T0251718

ENDOUROLOGY
A Practical Handbook

Uday Patel MBChB, MRCP, FRCP
Consultant Uroradiologist

Khurshid Ghani MBChB, BSc (Hons),
MRCS (Edin)
Endourology Research Fellow

Ken Anson MS, FRCS (Urol)
Consultant Urological Surgeon

St George's Hospital
London
UK

Foreword by
John EA Wickham and Michael J Kellett

informa
healthcare

New York London

First published in 2006 by Taylor & Francis, an imprint of the Taylor & Francis Group.
This edition published in 2011 by Informa Healthcare, Telephone House, 69-77 Paul Street, London EC2A 4LQ, UK.

Simultaneously published in the USA by Informa Healthcare, 52 Vanderbilt Avenue, 7th Floor, New York, NY 10017, USA.

Informa Healthcare is a trading division of Informa UK Ltd. Registered Office: 37–41 Mortimer Street, London W1T 3JH, UK. Registered in England and Wales number 1072954.

© 2006 Informa Healthcare, except as otherwise indicated

No claim to original U.S. Government works

Reprinted material is quoted with permission. Although every effort has been made to ensure that all owners of copyright material have been acknowledged in this publication, we would be glad to acknowledge in subsequent reprints or editions any omissions brought to our attention.

All rights reserved. No part of this publication may be reproduced, stored in a retrieval system, or transmitted, in any form or by any means, electronic, mechanical, photocopying, recording, or otherwise, unless with the prior written permission of the publisher or in accordance with the provisions of the Copyright, Designs and Patents Act 1988 or under the terms of any licence permitting limited copying issued by the Copyright Licensing Agency, 90 Tottenham Court Road, London W1P 0LP, UK, or the Copyright Clearance Center, Inc., 222 Rosewood Drive, Danvers, MA 01923, USA (http://www.copyright.com/ or telephone 978-750-8400).

Product or corporate names may be trademarks or registered trademarks, and are used only for identification and explanation without intent to infringe.

This book contains information from reputable sources and although reasonable efforts have been made to publish accurate information, the publisher makes no warranties (either express or implied) as to the accuracy or fitness for a particular purpose of the information or advice contained herein. The publisher wishes to make it clear that any views or opinions expressed in this book by individual authors or contributors are their personal views and opinions and do not necessarily reflect the views/opinions of the publisher. Any information or guidance contained in this book is intended for use solely by medical professionals strictly as a supplement to the medical professional's own judgement, knowledge of the patient's medical history, relevant manufacturer's instructions and the appropriate best practice guidelines. Because of the rapid advances in medical science, any information or advice on dosages, procedures, or diagnoses should be independently verified. This book does not indicate whether a particular treatment is appropriate or suitable for a particular individual. Ultimately it is the sole responsibility of the medical professional to make his or her own professional judgements, so as appropriately to advise and treat patients. Save for death or personal injury caused by the publisher's negligence and to the fullest extent otherwise permitted by law, neither the publisher nor any person engaged or employed by the publisher shall be responsible or liable for any loss, injury or damage caused to any person or property arising in any way from the use of this book.

A CIP record for this book is available from the British Library.

ISBN-13: 9781841843391

Orders may be sent to: Informa Healthcare, Sheepen Place, Colchester, Essex CO3 3LP, UK
Telephone: +44 (0)20 7017 5540
Email: CSDhealthcarebooks@informa.com
Website: http://informahealthcarebooks.com/

For corporate sales please contact: CorporateBooksIHC@informa.com
For foreign rights please contact: RightsIHC@informa.com
For reprint permissions please contact: PermissionsIHC@informa.com

CONTENTS

ILLUSTRATIONS

TABLES

FOREWORD

For ten years from 1969 to 1979 I was deeply involved with the problems presented by patients suffering from renal stone disease. Open stone surgery, particularly for the treatment of complicated staghorn calculi was traumatic. Hospital stay was usually seven to ten days with a six week convalescent period. For smaller stones particularly, such an approach often appeared to me unnecessarily interventionist.

In 1979 my very valued radiological colleague, Dr Michael Kellett who was at the Institute of Urology, London, was beginning to develop his skills with percutaneous needle puncture into the renal collecting system to relieve various obstructions.

Initially only fine tubes were inserted and in 1979 it became apparent to both of us that if the initial puncture tract could be dilated then it might be possible to insert an endoscope into the kidney, locate a small stone and even remove it. I believe it was in November of this year that a suitable patient presented with an 8.0 mm stone in a lower calyx. Accordingly Michael made a direct puncture into the kidney and using serial dilatation over a single wire increased the diameter of the tract to a size sufficient to allow me to pass a simple cystoscope into the kidney. I was then able to visualise the stone and by passing a Dornier basket down the operating channel, secure the stone and remove it. The patient was in hospital for two days and back to work within a week!

After this initial success it then became a matter of refining the process and developing more appropriate instrumentation with the help of the instrument manufacturers. As we attempted to treat larger stones it became necessary to develop access tracks which enabled the repeated passage of the endoscope and methods of fragmenting the calculi into removable pieces. These problems were finally solved by the application of plastic sheaths to maintain the track followed by the insertion of disintegratory instruments, ultrasound and electrohydraulic probes which could produce the necessary fragmentation: thus percutaneous nephrolithotomy became our standard form of treatment.

As is usual with such innovations, the same thought processes had occurred to other workers in various parts of the world, particularly Sweden and Germany and by 1983 a large volume of experience had been globally accumulated.

This experience was brought together in April of that year with the hosting of the first World Congress of Perctuneous Renal Surgery by the Institute of Urology in London when case reports of many hundreds of patients so treated were presented.

Following this a teaching programme commenced at the Institute with practical demonstrations and hands on courses conducted biannually, admirably organised by Ron Miller.

In the same year Eisenburger in Germany advanced the introduction of extracorporeal shockwave lithotripsy which rapidly superseded percutaneous stone surgery as the principal method of management of most stones, however percutaneous intrarenal surgery still remains a most necessary adjunct to the treatment of larger calculi.

The learning curve for Urologists and Radiologists performing percutaneous manipulations in the urinary tract should be considerably shortened by consulting this highly informative text. We would very much commend this book as a valuable and necessary guide to the skills required by anyone who assumes to provide a comprehensive armamentarium for the treatment of patients with renal stone disease.

In a decade we and many other workers were enabled to completely change the outlook for patients suffering with renal stone from a very unpleasant traumatic event to what has in most cases become a walk-in walk-out procedure. As an added bonus for us it was a most exciting and fulfilling experience.

John E A Wickham, Michael J Kellett

ACKNOWLEDGEMENTS

We would like to thank all theatre staff, radiographers and anaesthetists who allowed their photos to be used, and Boston Scientific for assistance with equipment pictures. We would like to thank all our patients who consented to be photographed and all our trainers who have taught us over the years. Finally we would like to thank our families for their unstinting support.

'I will not covet persons labouring under the stone, but will leave this to be done by men who are practitioners of this craft'

Hippocratic Oath

PART I
EQUIPMENT AND TECHNICAL DETAILS

1. BASIC ENDOSCOPIC PRINCIPLES

INTRODUCTION

The modern day endourologist has an extraordinary array of instruments and ancillary gadgets at his disposal that could only have been dreamt about 15 years ago and could not possibly have been conceived 30 years ago. A patient presenting in the new millennium with a ureteric or renal calculus can realistically anticipate full stone clearance either by extracorporeal techniques or by minimally invasive endoscopic alternatives that will not require an incision and can be performed with predictably low morbidity. There have been remarkable developments in the technique of lithotomy from the itinerant lithotomists of the nineteenth century (Figure 1.1) to the modern day stone surgeon. This has only become possible from the coming together of industrial expertise with urologists to develop ever-smaller diagnostic endoscopes and therapeutic ancillary instruments. Each new revolution in endoscopic design has allowed access to more remote areas of the genitourinary system

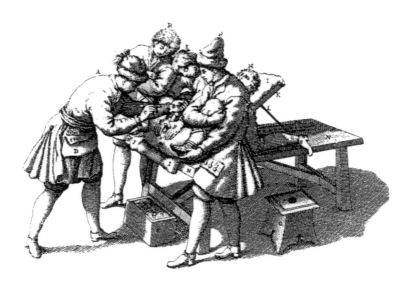

Figure 1.1 Stone surgery in the nineteenth century.

and although initially diagnoses were eminently feasible, therapeutic options were limited. Miniaturisation of the therapeutic instruments has initially lagged behind endoscopic design, but our manufacturing colleagues have usually caught up. As a result the revolution in endoscopic management of bladder lesions that occurred toward the end of the last century is now being repeated in the treatment of pelvicalyceal pathologies.

In this chapter we will outline the basic generic principles that govern endourology techniques from rigid urethroscopy to flexible ureterorenoscopy. The specific techniques applicable for each procedure will be listed in the relevant chapter. Laparoscopic procedures are beyond the remit of this textbook.

ENDOSCOPE DESIGN

Our pioneering predecessors performed the original endoscopies with single metal tubes with either candles or small light bulbs attached to the proximal end. Indeed, some used light reflected by face mirrors, as still being used by our ear, nose and throat (ENT) colleagues (Figure 1.2). The image quality must have been extremely poor (however perhaps endourologists of the future will think similarly of our modern day techniques!). The development of the rod lens system by Hopkins in the late 1940s changed everything and enabled light to be transmitted to the end of the endoscope, thus illuminating the lumen of interest and simultaneously allowing transmission of the image from the end of the endoscope to the eyepiece of the scope for viewing. Many of our lower tract endoscopes today still employ this technology and have changed little in design over the last 50 years.

The rigid ureteroscope was introduced in the 1970s and these are now available in sizes ranging from 4.5 to 11.5F (measured at the tip). Most increase in size from the tip to the shaft of the instrument (Figure 1.3) and one must be aware of this as commonly navigation of the instrument in the ureter is limited by the wider proximal shaft being 'held up' at the vesicoureteric junction. The instruments used today range in size from 6.0 to 8.5 F and are so-called semi-rigid endoscopes due to the minor flexibility of the metallic shaft. They commonly employ fibreoptic technology rather than the rod lens systems.

The introduction of fibreoptics in the 1960s led to the next revolution in endoscope design. Fibreoptic fibres are gathered together to produce cables that can be incorporated into endoscopes as image and light bundles. The

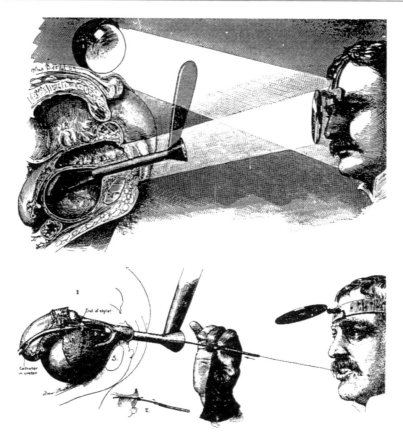

Figure 1.2 Early cystoscopy.

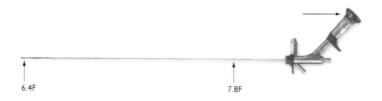

6.4F   7.8F

Figure 1.3 Standard semirigid ureteroscopy design. This scope is 45 cm long with an angled eyepiece (arrow) to allow rigid instruments to be delivered into the working channel. The tip of the scope is 6.4F which increases to 7.8F proximally. (Courtesy of KeyMed Olympus)

flexibility of these bundles has led to the development of flexible endoscopes (Figure 1.4), which are steerable and fully flexible through 360° with limited loss of image quality. Further advances in fibreoptic technology have led to increased miniaturisation of the bundles allowing the present day flexible

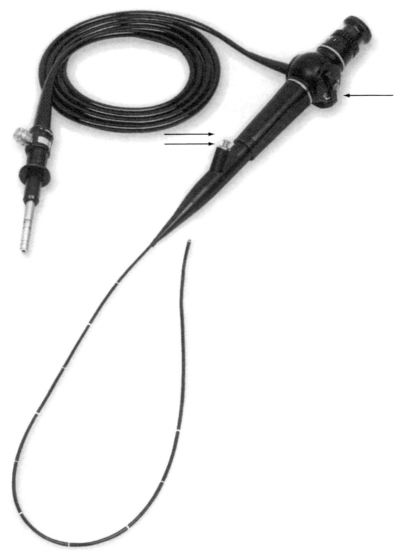

Figure 1.4 Standard flexible ureterorenoscopy design. This scope is 70 cm in length with a flexible tip controlled by the deflector lever (arrow). Instruments and/or irrigation are delivered via the 3.6 Fr single working channel (double arrows). (Courtesy of KeyMed Olympus)

6.8 Fr ureterorenoscope (URS) to incorporate a 3.6 Fr instrument channel whilst also being steerable with nearly one to one torque and 270° deflection. These have brought the whole of the pelvicalyceal system into diagnostic and therapeutic range for the modern endourologist.

LIGHT SOURCES

Light is required at the end of the endoscope to illuminate the field of view. It should be of an intensity to allow the whole field to be illuminated to allow sufficient light to be reflected back via the image bundle for viewing 'downstream'. Initially standard tungsten-halogen bulbs were used, but the advent of the xenon light source has considerably improved the illumination of endoscopes. These are now the light sources of choice throughout the world. Xenon light sources are very powerful and are essential when dealing with video endoscopy and the reduced light transmission of fine flexible endoscopes.

The light source is connected to the endoscope via a flexible, fibreoptic cable. The efficiency of light transmission is reduced as the cable length increases. Modern light sources are usually incorporated into complex camera systems that provide feedback to the light source on the amount of light at the business end of the endoscope. The light source automatically adjusts its intensity, allowing sufficient light to be available in dark recesses, and reduces glare when coming up close to tissues (automatic brightness control). They are small, compact units that may also incorporate intensity-mode memories, standby illumination modes (to improve the lifetime of the bulbs) and spare bulbs that can cut in as soon as required.

> DON'T! Old light guide cables with multiple broken fibres can be the weak link in the chain and let down the most expensive endoscope and camera system

The recent introduction of blue light illumination has generated great interest in the diagnosis of subtle premalignant conditions in the gastrointestinal tract and bronchial tree. When combined with a fluorescence agent such as amino laevulinic acid (ALA) it is said to have a greater sensitivity and specificity for carcinoma *in situ* of the bladder over conventional white light cystoscopy.

INSTRUMENT CHANNELS

The final element of an endoscope design is the instrument channel. This allows both the influx and efflux of irrigant solution, the delivery of ancillary devices to the operative field and for aspiration of urine and irrigant for sampling. All endoscope designs aim to provide as large an instrument channel as possible in order to offer the greatest range of therapeutic options available. With the use of optical fibres, modern day instruments can incorporate instrument channels as large as 75% of the overall diameter of the endoscopes. Recently this has allowed channels large enough to accommodate both a grasping device and ballistic energy probe into the single channel. Also the most recent semirigid ureteroscope designs incorporate two separate channels allowing so-called 'continuous flow' irrigation to take place (Figure 1.5). This provides the option to keep one channel permanently open, thus balancing hydrostatic pressure within the ureter during endoscopy and the drainage of the 'snow storm' that follows laser lithotripsy and fine fragmentation of ureteric calculi.

Knowledge of the diameter of the instrument channel of each endoscope available is vital to the success of therapeutic endoscopy as suitable instruments can then be chosen for the task at hand. In addition, a balance can be struck between the largest diameter device available and the amount of space left for the irrigant influx to maintain adequate views.

Finally the instrument channel needs to be protected when delivering devices along it, particularly with flexible endoscopes. The channel itself can be damaged and 'rucked up', particularly by sharp instruments such as laser fibres. At this point there is also a danger of damage to the deflecting wires if the instrument is forced onward against resistance.

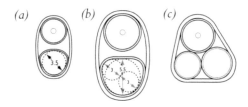

Figure 1.5 Cross-section of the tip of a ureteroscope demonstrating relationship of the optics (o) to a number of instrument channel designs available. (a) Single channel (3.5F), (b) single channel (5.5F), or two channels (3F each), (c) triangular sheath with two channels (2.4 and 3.4F). (Courtesy of KeyMed Olympus)

DON'T! Instruments can be damaged if delivered down a deflected scope

OPTICAL LINK

The image can be reflected from the operating field to the eyepiece via either the rodlens system or fibre optics. A recent innovation is to place a charge-coupled device (CCD) at the tip of the endoscope. This device digitises the image and transmits it via internal wires to the CCD processor, thus obviating the need for an external camera. The vast majority of the endoscopes in use today use the rodlens or fibreoptic system in which the image is either viewed directly at the eyepiece or detected by a camera (incorporating a single or multiple CCDs) attached to the eyepiece. The image is then manipulated at the CCD processing unit and transmitted to the monitor (Figure 1.6). Clearly many different problems can affect the quality of the image visualised by the surgeon and some of these are listed in Table 1.1. A confident, ordered approach to troubleshooting should lead to rapid resolution of the problem.

> DON'T! A confused random approach to image problems only leads to more confusion, frustration, delay and unhappiness!

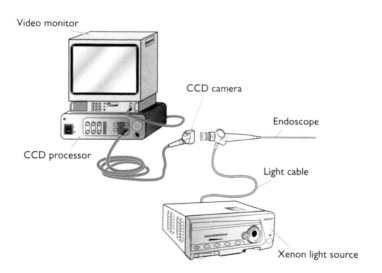

Figure 1.6 Illustration demonstrating the set-up of the endoscope to the light source, camera and monitor. (Courtesy of KeyMed Olympus)

Table 1.1 How to approach image problems during surgery

Image	Problem	Action
No image	Incorrect connection	Check power
	Loose connection	Check all connections
	Faulty kit	
Cloudy	Wet interface	Dry camera and eyepiece
	Camera cover sitting between camera and eyepiece	Remove plastic cover Check endoscope not faulty by direct vision
Blurred	Poor focus	Correct camera focus
		Correct endoscope focus
		Check endoscope not faulty by direct vision
Glare	Too much light	Check automatic brightness control is on
		If so go to manual and adjust
		Alter iris setting
Poor colour reproduction	Incorrect balance	White balance camera with each endoscope used
		Check monitor colour settings

INTUBATION AND NAVIGATION

A few guiding principles govern all endoscopic manipulations irrespective of the organ being studied. Often intubation of the orifice is the most awkward part of the endoscopy and this is certainly true of ureteroscopy. Lubrication of the endoscope aids movement and accommodation of the orifice, but if intubation cannot be achieved without pushing then dilatation of that orifice may be necessary. Before the recent development of smaller ureteroscopes (<8–9F) ureteric dilatation was considered necessary to allow intubation and to prevent damage to the vesicoureteric junction. Often post-operative oedema at the orifice after dilatation results in considerable post-operative morbidity and hence ureteric stenting is indicated if the orifice is dilated. However, the narrow ureteroscopes can now be passed comfortably and post-endoscopic stenting is not routinely required.

Following intubation the endoscope needs to be navigated to the area of interest or to explore the full extent of the organ. The instrument should be advanced gently and slowly with soft hands and loose wrists. This allows the natural contours of the organ to direct the endoscope rather than the surgeon trying to manipulate the anatomy to fit.

> DO! The lumen should be kept in the middle of the screen at all times.

If the lumen is tangential on the screen it is likely that part of the endoscope will be pressed against the lumen wall with potential for damage. If the lumen appears to take an awkward direction ahead then you can use fluoroscopy to define the exact anatomy before attempting to negotiate it. One should attempt to adopt a field view of the whole image available and look into the far field as much as in the near field (much as one looks into the distance whilst driving rather than concentrating on the boot of the car in front).

> DON'T! The most important guiding principle for endoscopic naviga-tion is not to push.

If resistance is significant and the endoscope is forced ahead, permanent damage can result from perforation/ischaemic compression or worst of all detachment of the organ from its attachments (i.e ureter from bladder or kidney!). Often trainees ask how much can one push and the answer is always the same – if any resistance is encountered, stop! Experienced endoscopists do, however, occasionally push, but this is performed with other factors being taken into account. Some peripheral clues are available to help (move-ment of the scope in relation to both the safety wire and lumen wall is re-assuring and fluoroscopy can help to confirm safe transit of the scope). If in doubt stop and come back another day or perform dilatation by another controlled method.

The endoscope can be passed over a guidewire that has already been suc-cessfully placed in the area of interest. The advantage of this approach is that the scope should reach the destination with minimal trauma, however having reached the target area there will be no space in the instrument channel for any therapeutic instruments. The endoscope will need to be removed from the wire and passed alongside or the guide wire can then be removed leaving the channel fully available (our preferred method for flexible ureterorenoscopy). An alternative is to pass the scope alongside a safety wire using it as a guide by keeping it in view throughout the navigation (our preferred method for semirigid ureteroscopy).

Hydrostatic irrigant pressure can also be of value during navigation but beware of air bubbles in the system (Figure 1.7). A gentle temporary rise in the height of the irrigation solution can passively distend the lumen sufficiently to allow the endoscope through. Alternatively, either squeezing the bag or using a syringe loaded with saline via the instrument channel can apply some extra pressure. A useful recent addition to the armamentarium is a foot-operated syringe driver, which frees up both hands to manipulate the endoscope and any ancillary instruments.

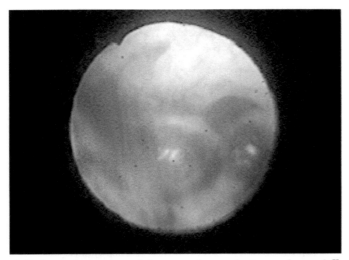

Figure 1.7 *Air in the ureter or kidney can distort the image due to diffraction at the air/fluid interface.*

DO! Reduce the pressure as soon as the endoscope has been navigated through the difficult area in order to prevent end organ endoscopic hydrostatic pressure damage

THEATRE ENVIRONMENT

The theatre set up is crucial to the success of all endoscopic surgery. The patient must be positioned comfortably on a radiograph-compatible table allowing access to the parts of the body that require screening during the procedure. The surgeon must be comfortable with the position of all staff and equipment in the theatre in order to ensure success. There must be ample room for the surgeon and assistant, the scrub nurse, the radiographer and image intensifier, the endoscopic stack and monitors, energy sources required, ancillary instrument trays and, of course, the anaesthetist, anaesthetic machine and trolleys. All this should be in a theatre regularly used for the purpose so that all the necessary ancillary endoscopic and disposable instruments are rapidly to hand and not five minutes down the corridor. It is the nature of this sort of surgery that the unexpected often does happen and the 'kitchen sink' should be available at all times.

SUGGESTED FURTHER READING

Whitfield HN, Gupta SK. Urological Instrumentation. In Mundy AR, Neal D, George NJR, Fitzpatrick J, eds. Scientific Basis of Urology, 2nd edn. London: Martin Dunitz, 2004

2. PRINCIPLES OF IMAGING IN ENDOUROLOGY

An endourologist needs to be familiar with many aspects of the imaging modalities as they are as indispensable as the endoscope (Box 2.1). A thorough understanding of their underlying principles are essential to gain maximum advantage from these techniques, and also to ensure the necessary margin of safety for both the patient and the operator.

Box 2.1 Imaging modalities used in endourology (in order of frequency)

- Plain radiography
- Intravenous urography
- Fluoroscopy
- Ultrasound
- Nuclear medicine
- Computerised tomography
- Magnetic resonance tomography

PLAIN RADIOGRAPHY

The plain radiograph of the kidneys, ureter and bladder (KUB), still retains a vital role in endourology. Traditional radiographic film (the silver halide film) is still unsurpassed in depiction of fine detail. Fine calcification is most easily appreciated on this film and especially with tomography (Figure 2.1). In current practice the plain radiograph is most useful for the initial investigation of suspected renal calculi and follow-up of known renal and particularly ureteric calculi (Box 2.2).

Compared with computerised tomography (CT) as the reference standard, KUB has a low sensitivity for diagnosing calculi (range 45–58%). Stones may be radiolucent, whilst body habitus and bowel gas or faeces may obscure.

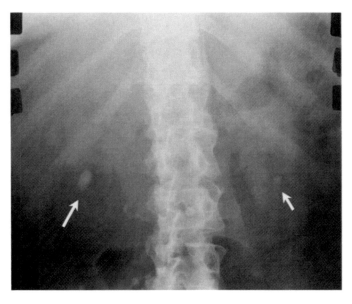

Figure 2.1 A plain radiograph showing bilateral renal calculi (arrowed).

Box 2.2 Plain radiograph (the KUB film)

- Good for follow-up of ureteral calculi
- Radiation dose is around 1 mSv (or 50 times that of a CXR)
- Some calculi are radiolucent (e.g. uric acid, struvite)

DO! A KUB must be available when planning intervention or identifying the movement of radio-opaque stone fragments after intervention

INTRAVENOUS UROGRAPHY

Intravenous urography (IVU) is the workhorse imaging modality in endourology. It is good for diagnostic assessment and also provides reliable spatial, anatomical and functional information. Endoscopic navigation is closely dependent on the operator having a mental picture of directions and ramifications of the ureter and upper urinary tract. This can be appreciated from a good quality IVU (Figure 2.2). The disadvantages of the IVU are its higher radiation dose, the necessity for intravenous contrast media and that

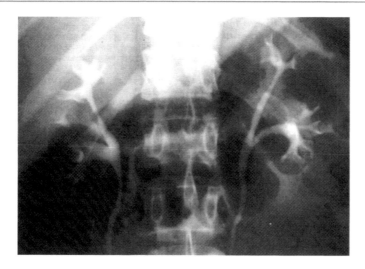

Figure 2.2 An IVU image showing good global representation of upper tract anatomy.

it is limited to a two-dimensional format – any three-dimensional information is assumed (for example the orientation of the calyces, whether anterior
or posterior). Nevertheless, the IVU is still the most widely used modality
for global evaluation of the urinary tract (Box 2.3).

Box 2.3 The intravenous urogram

Advantages

- Global diagnostic and anatomical information for endourological
  planning
- Information easily assimilated
- Readily available

Disadvantages

- Radiation 2–3 times annual background radiation (between 3 to 4.5
  msv)
- Radiolucent stones poorly seen
- Renal toxic iodinated contrast media necessary

DO! An IVU should be available for PCNL planning

> **DON'T!** Use an IVU and KUB indiscriminately. Those with stable stone disease can be followed up using renal ultrasound alone

> **DO!** With a female patient, make sure there is no likelihood of pregnancy before any radiation use

IODINATED CONTRAST MEDIA

Only a sufficient density gradient between adjacent tissues will confer radiographic visibility, for example calcium-containing stones or bones are easily seen, but the fluid-containing renal calyces and pelvis cannot be differentiated from surrounding renal parenchyma on a plain abdominal radiograph. Radiographic contrast media (CM) are oral or intravenous agents able to accentuate the natural tissue density gradients, and so enhance radiographic visibility. The currently used intravenous contrast agents are iodine (atomic weight 127) containing compounds designed to be hydrophilic, with low lipid solubility or protein binding, and with molecular weights <2000. This ensures brisk dissemination into the extravascular, extracellular space and rapid excretion. All body soft tissues enhance, and the kidneys particularly so as they are the principal source of excretion (99%) with a half-life of 2 hours. CM further undergo 50–100-fold concentration within the kidney and so are an ideal agent for the study of upper tract and ureteric anatomy. The down side is the various adverse effects of CM and these are listed in Box 2.4.

Box 2.4 Adverse reactions to iodinated radiographic contrast media

---

- Nausea and vomiting
- Rigors
- Sneezing
- Urticaria
- Bronchospasm
- Vagal reactions
- Contrast media nephrotoxicity
- Anaphylactoid reactions (angio-oedema, laryngeal oedema, bronchospasm, circulatory collapse)

The most modern agents are now iso-osmolar and have lower toxicity. However, some patients may be at a high risk of an adverse reaction. Box 2.5 details the management of these patients.

> DO! Consider contrast-related risks: previous contrast reaction or allergic history, diabetes mellitus (on metformin), renal disease and NSAIDs are all risk factors

Box 2.5 Management of patients at a high risk of contrast reaction

High risk of allergic reaction

- Patients with a previous history of reaction to contrast medium, iodine allergy (allergy to topical iodine is not a risk factor), severe seafood allergy, history of anaphylaxis are high-risk groups
- Those with a severe previous reaction (e.g. anaphylactic shock, angioneurotic oedema, etc.) should not receive iodinated contrast media
- Those with less severe reactions in the past (e.g. rash, itching, etc.) can have iodinated contrast medium after steroid prophylaxis (e.g. predinosolone 10 mg qid for 24 hours before)
- Those having ureterography alone should be treated along the same lines as there is a risk of intravasation during this procedure

High risk of renal toxicity

- Patients with existing renal disease, diabetes mellitus, non-steroidal drug therapy, etc., are a high-risk group
- Renal toxicity is higher if the creatinine level is >200 mg/l
- Iodinated contrast media should be avoided
- If i.v. contrast medium is used the following are said to reduce renal impairment:
  a) Intravenous saline (100 ml/hr for 24 hours)
  b) Metformin should be stopped
  c) Oral acetylcysteine (although this is disputed by some)
- Ureterography has no significant risk. No special measures necessary other than avoiding extravasation

DO! Stop Metformin 48 hours before and after CM investigation in order to avoid renal failure and lactic acidosis. Check blood chemistry before restarting Metformin

FLUOROSCOPY

This is real-time radiography and is essential for both percutaneous nephrolithotomy (PCNL) and ureterorenoscopy. The image is viewed on a TV monitor and is not as sharp as a plain radiograph but is 'live', and by rotating the fluoroscopic arm, the spatial relationships between structures are appreciated (this principle is further covered in Chapter 5). This facility is particularly exploited when a PCNL track is being created. Box 2.6 explains the technique of fluoroscopy.

Box 2.6 Fluoroscopy during endourology

- Always maintain the area of interest in the centre of the field as it will be seen sharpest
- Give clear instructions to the radiographer
- Contrast injection – usually dilute contrast (1:1 or 1:2) is best, as stones will not be masked. However, in some situations neat agents are better, e.g. when investigating papillary necrosis, or with an obese patient.
    - (a) Inject contrast slowly to avoid extravasation
    - (b) Avoid air bubbles, this may be confused with filling defects or may act as an 'air block'
- Record any abnormalities (but to reduce the radiation dose to the patient ask the radiographer to 'capture' or 'store' the fluoroscopic image)

DO! Bony or bowel shadow may be confused as ureteric abnormalities. Rotating the c arm will help evaluation of suspected artefacts

During all circumstances, fluoroscopy (Figure 2.3) should be used judiciously to minimise the radiation burden to both the patient and the

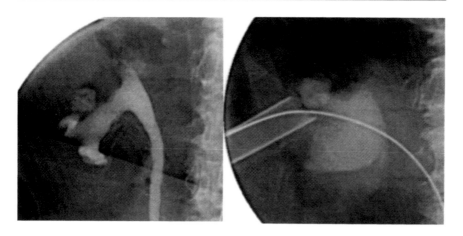

Figure 2.3 A fluoroscopic stored image taken during PCNL.

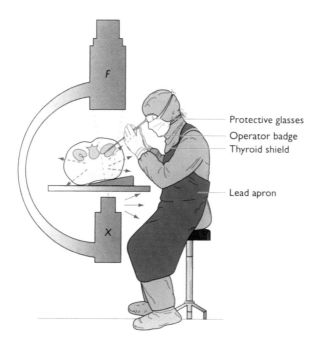

Protective glasses
Operator badge
Thyroid shield

Lead apron

Figure 2.4 A line drawing showing how radiation may reach the patient and operator during PCNL. The red lines show the path of direct radiation reaching the operator from the source (X) and the hatched lines represent indirect or scattered radiation. Box 2.7 lists how the radiation dose may be minimised.

operator. Radiation reaches either directly from the tube generator or via scattered rays. Figure 2.4 demonstrates the working position of the endourologist and the various ways radiation may reach him/her, and Box 2.7 summarises how the radiation dose can be minimised.

Box 2.7 Reducing the radiation dose during endourological procedures

To the patient

- Use minimal exposure
- Use capture facility rather than full exposures
- Collimate beam tightly
- Have the C-arm as close to the patient as possible
- Take your foot off the pedal when not in use!

To the operator

- All of the above
- Use lead shielding (at least 0.35 mm thick lead apron). Consider using thyroid shield and lead glasses
- Keep hands out of the primary beam (angling the beam away allows working without hands in the beam, but this increases scatter dose to the operator)
- Stay as far away from the radiation source as possible (radiation obeys the inverse square law in air)
- Monitor dose received with a film badge

DO! Use fluoroscopy carefully, as the radiation dose can easily build up

---

RADIATION USE DURING PREGNANCY

The radiation damage to the growing fetus includes malformation, growth retardation, carcinogenesis and genetic defects. The first two of this group occur once a threshold is exceeded (thought to be >50 mGy) while the last two have no threshold and become more probable with increasing dose. The risks to the growing fetus from a limited IVU (assuming the radiation dose is limited to 2 mGy) of fatal or non-fatal cancer is 1:16 500 and the risk of heritable disease is 1:21 000. There is no added risk from the use of iodinated contrast media in pregnancy. As far as possible radiation should be avoided, and the use of ultrasound and modern MRI can resolve most cases of suspected acute colic during pregnancy. If intervention is necessary then nephrostomy can be carried out under ultrasound guidance alone and retrograde stenting and ureteroscopy can be carried out without the use of fluoroscopy in many cases. If necessary, very limited fluoroscopy with careful shielding of the uterus can be carried out after proper patient counselling.

ULTRASOUND

Ultrasound is the safest and most versatile imaging modality (Figure 2.5). In the urinary tract its particular advantage is that all stones, regardless of their make-up, are visible as long as they are large enough (the only exception being certain drug-induced calculi, such as those secondary to indinavir) and that it is a real-time modality that can be used for needle puncture and intervention. Ultrasound is unrivalled for the acute management of urinary stone disease with excellent sensitivity for diagnosing hydronephrosis. The accuracy of stone diagnosis is dependent on the size and the location of the stone. The overall sensitivity for detecting calculi ranges from 37% to 64%. Small stones are less likely to produce an acoustic shadow and are difficult to diagnose. Stones in the pelvicalyceal system can be reliably identified only if they are larger than 5 mm. Stones in the ureter are rarely visualised unless they are within the proximal ureter. The advantages and shortcomings are summarised in Box 2.8.

Box 2.8 Ultrasound in endourology

Advantages

- Safe
- Real time
- All stones (except indinavir, and struvite) are visible
- Can be used to guide PCNL puncture

Disadvantages

- Operator dependent
- Ureters not visualised
- Upper tract TCCs may not be clearly seen
- Air (that may be introduced during endoscopy) may be mistaken for calculus
- 3D capability still rudimentary

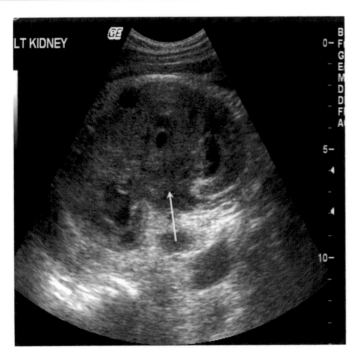

Figure 2.5 An ultrasound image of the left kidney showing the calyces and pelvis entirely replaced by soft tissue mass (arrow) that proved to be tumour.

> DO! Ultrasonography can be useful for diagnosing stones at the vesicoureteric junction (VUJ), an area that can be difficult to visualize on KUB

COMPUTERISED TOMOGRAPHY IN ENDOUROLOGY

The advent of spiral CT in the mid 1990s had a major impact on our ability to diagnose renal and ureteric calculi. This was particularly so with acute colic and the recognition of small obstructing ureteric calculi. It is now recognised that the traditional modalities of plain radiography and ultrasound miss many stones. Non-contrast helical CT (NCHCT) is the most accurate modality for the evaluation of acute colic and comparative data are summarised in Box 2.9. More than 99% of stones, including those that are radiolucent on KUB, will be seen when NCHCT is used. Pure matrix stones and stones made of indinavir, a human immunodeficiency virus protease inhibitor, are the exceptions. Further advantages of NCHCT over an IVU are that it does not require intravenous contrast injection and is a very rapid investigation.

Box 2.9 Stone diagnosis: accuracy compared to NCHCT

- KUB is 45–75% accurate
- IVU is 85% accurate
- US is now thought to be only 25–30% accurate

Another advantage of CT is that it is an accurate representation of anatomical relationships, and the most modern machines offer the possibility of fine and faithful three-dimensional (3D) reconstruction (Box 2.10, Figure 2.6). Such information has the potential to revolutionise endoscopic navigation and treatment. The disadvantage is that the radiation dose is two to three times greater than that imparted by a standard IVU, and this will limit the greater application of CT in endourology. Magnetic resonance imaging has the potential to offer all these advantages and more, without any radiation burden, but requires further technical developments before it can match the capability of CT.

(a)

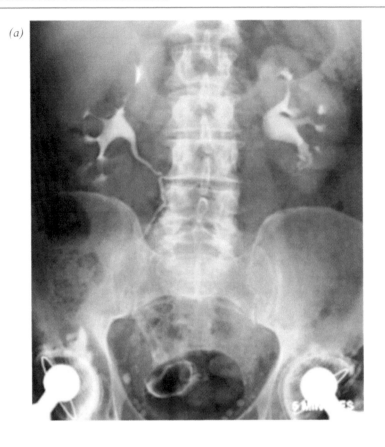

(b)

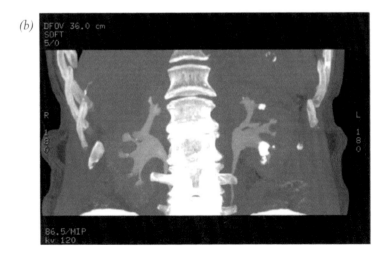

(c)

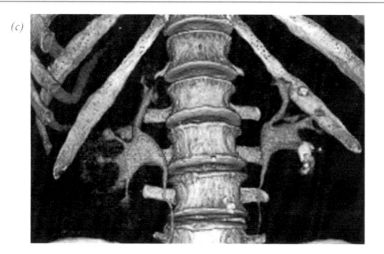

Figure 2.6 A montage showing an IVU (a) and two different CT urography representations of the upper tract anatomy and stones in the lower pole of the left kidney. The first CT image (b) is a coronal reconstruction and the second (c) a 3D volume rendered reconstruction. Modern 3D CT can provide the most complete and accurate representation of urinary tract stones and anatomy.

Box 2.10 Advantages and disadvantages of CT

Advantages

- High diagnostic accuracy
- Faithful anatomical and spatial reconstruction
- Best for pre-operative PCNL planning

Disadvantages

- Cost
- High radiation burden
- Fixed, non-mobile units
- Limited availability

NUCLEAR MEDICINE

Nuclear medicine renal scans can be used to define the percentage contribution of each kidney to global renal function (the Dimercaptosuccine acid (DMSA) or Mercaptoacetyl-glycine (MAG 3) scan) or objectively study the drainage characteristics of a kidney (the DTPA or MAG 3 scans) (Figure 2.7). Both sets of information are very useful for patient evaluation and for directing management. For example, a kidney with a staghorn calculus and only 10% preserved function (after any associated infection is treated) is probably not worth treating by PCNL as stone clearance is unlikely to improve function sufficiently.

Regarding post-procedure function, numerous studies have demonstrated that PCNL (and Extracorporeal shockwave lithotripsy (ESWL)) have no deleterious effect with good preservation of long-term renal function, as measured by nuclear medicine or creatinine clearance.

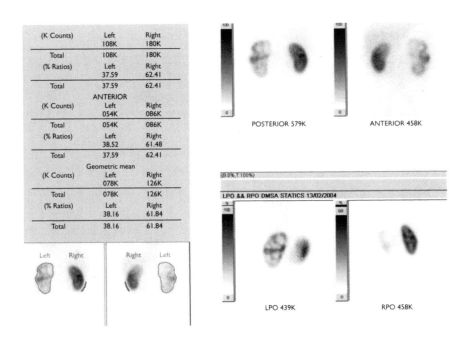

Figure 2.7 This is a Nuclear Medicine scan (DMSA) showing reduced function of the left kidney secondary to a large staghorn calculus. Assessment of residual renal function of a stone bearing kidney can help to decide whether the kidney is not worth salvaging as it has lost too much function already, and nephrectomy is more appropriate.

DO! Consider a renal scan prior to embarking on major stone surgery as the kidney may already have lost most of its function

SUGGESTED FURTHER READING

European Society of Uroradiology. Guidelines on the use of contrast media. http://www.esur.org/guidelines.cfm

Grainger RG, Allison DJ. Diagnostic Radiology – A Textbook of Medical Imaging, 4th edn. London: Churchill Livingstone, 1997

Khoo L, Anson KM, Patel U. Success and short-term complication rates of percutaneous nephrostomy during pregnancy. J Vasc Interv Radiol 2004; 15: 1469–73

Lee JKT, Sagel SS, Stanley RJ, Heiken JP. Computed Tomography with MRI correlation, 3rd edn. New York: Raven Press, 1998

Patel U. Principles of uroradiology. In Mundy AR, Neal D, George NJR, Fitzpatrick J, eds. Scientific Basis of Urology, 2nd edn. London: Martin Dunitz, 2004

Sandhu C, Anson KM, Patel U. Urinary tract stones – part I: role of radiological imaging in diagnosis and treatment planning. Clin Radiol 2003; 58: 415–21

3. Equipment used in Endourology

Like many modern surgical specialties, endourology is much dependent on the array of specialised equipment available. Over the 30 years or so since the specialty began there have been many refinements in equipment with accompanying improvements in the success and safety of the various endourological procedures. Although the range of equipment available and used is wide, some items can be considered basic to the specialty. Knowledge of these items and their functional principles is essential background knowledge for the endourologist. These are detailed in Box 3.1 and for descriptive order they are considered under the broad subgroups of disposable and non-disposable (or re-usable) equipment.

Box 3.1 Disposable and non-disposable equipment in endourology

Disposables	Non-disposables
• Guidewires	• Metal dilators
• Retrieval devices	• Intracorporeal lithotriptors
• Stents/catheters	• Endoscopes
• Balloons and dilators	

DISPOSABLE EQUIPMENT

Wires and their use

A landmark moment in minimally invasive procedures was Lunderquist's description of the use of a guidewire to support the percutaneous insertion of a catheter. Without a guidewire it is impossible to envisage any endourological procedure and a thorough understanding of guidewires is fundamental to successful endourological practice. Inserted under fluoroscopic control, guidewires help gain and maintain access within the urinary tract (Box 3.2). Many types of wires are available differentiated by their material of composition, size, tip design, shaft rigidity, surface coating and length. Thorough knowledge of the different structural properties allows the appropriate guidewire to be chosen for the task in hand, saving time and increasing the chances of operative success.

Box 3.2 Functions of a guidewire

- Access: gains retrograde/antegrade access to the upper urinary tract
- Structure: conforms rigidity and straightens the course of the ureter
- Guide: helps passage of endoscopes, stents and catheters
- Safety: maintains access to the organ of interest during procedures

---

Structural properties

Size

Wires can range in diameter from 0.018 (1.4F) to 0.038 inch (2.9F) and 80 to 260 cm in length. The average working length of a guidewire for upper tract endoscopy is 150 cm, and a diameter of 0.035–0.038 inch is ideal (Figure 3.1).

Tip

Tips vary in their length, shape and flexibility. All wires have a distal tip that is soft and flexible (floppy) for easier and less traumatic passage through the

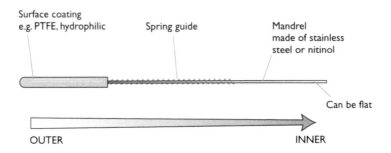

Figure 3.1 Schematic representation of the structure of a guidewire. The standard working wire is a 0.038 inch polytetrafluoroethylene (PTFE) coated 145 cm guidewire with a 3 cm straight floppy tip.

ureter – a floppy tip will bounce off the wall of the ureter rather than puncture through or dissect the wall and raise a flap. The standard floppy tip is 3 cm in length, but this can vary from 3 to 15 cm. The choice of length of the floppy end is little more than personal preference, but a long floppy tip is difficult to control when used to probe an opening, e.g. the ureteral orifice. The standard wire has a soft and hard or stiff end, but wires with a floppy tip on each end are used for flexible ureterorenoscopy to allow easy backloading into the working channel of the endoscope. Various tip shapes are available to help overcome difficult ureteral intubation or tortuous ureteral anatomy (Table 3.1 and Figure 3.2).

Shaft rigidity

A guidewire consists of an inner metal core (mandrel) which is covered by a tightly coiled thin spring wire (spring guide) (Figure 3.1). The spring guide acts as a track for the smooth passage of endoscopes or catheters. The size and stiffness of the mandrel determine the rigidity and strength of the wire.

Material of composition

Most wires have a mandrel made of stainless steel, which may be round or flat in cross-section. Round wires have a standard stiffness. Flat wires are used in stiff wires, as they provide greater rigidity without a further increase

Table 3.1 Different guidewire tips and their uses

Straight	J tip	Angled
• Most normal conditions	• Helps prevents ureteral perforation in delicate ureter	• Helps intubate eccentrically located ureteric orifice
• Try this first	• Useful for impacted calculi	• Helps with tortuous ureter
	• Ureteral tortuosity	• Useful for probing total obstructions

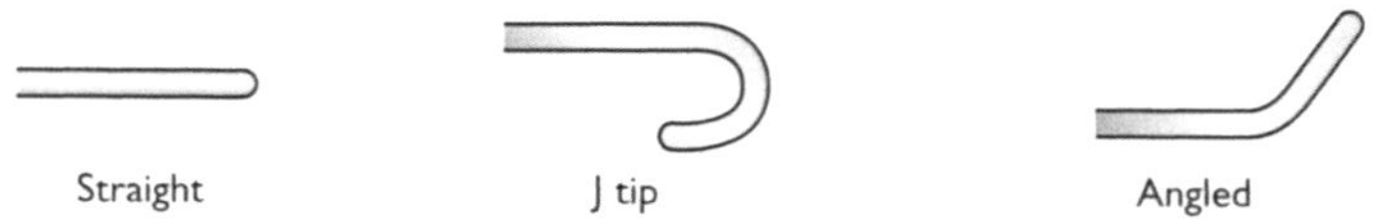

Straight   J tip   Angled

Figure 3.2 Different types of guidewire tips.

in the overall diameter. The mandrel may be removable but most are fixed wires with a mandrel made of nitinol as described in Box 3.3.

Box 3.3 Nitinol wires

Recently wires have been developed with a mandrel made of nickel titanium alloy, otherwise known as nitinol (an acronym of NIckel TItanium Naval Ordinance Laboratory). Unlike stainless steel, these wires are kink resistant and can be designed with a stiffer core (e.g. Glidewire®, Boston Scientific). They also have 'memory', allowing it to coil and recoil

---

Coating

The frictional resistance of a guidewire is determined by its stiffness and coefficient of friction. The coefficient of resistance depends on the surface characteristics. The coating reduces friction along the surface. The standard surface coating of a guidewire is PTFE (Teflon®). Compared to steel, PTFE reduces the coefficient of friction by half, whilst the friction coefficient of hydrophilic wires is only one-sixth that of stainless steel. PTFE offers a smooth surface for easy passage through the urinary tract and improves the advancement of rigid devices. It keeps its place within the ureter and does not slip out.

Box 3.4 Hydrophilic polymer coated wires

These wires have a much lower coefficient of friction than PTFE wires, and permit near frictionless passage (e.g. Terumo Glidewire, Boston Scientific or the Roadrunner wire, Cook). They are particularly useful for negotiating past an impacted calculus or a tortuous ureter, or for probing total obstructions. These wires are suitable for softer devices. However, the very properties that allow easy passage also mean that dissection of the ureteral wall can be easily created

---

Hybrid wires

Recently manufacturers have started producing heterogeneous wires fit for most purposes. They are more expensive and consist of different segments coated with different materials such that all the major needs of endoscopic surgery are fulfilled in one wire, e.g. Sensor™ (Microvasive, Boston Scientific). The Sensor™ is made of a distal hydrophilic tip with a nitinol PTFE-coated body (Figure 3.3). The tip is slippery enough to negotiate past an impacted stone and the nitinol body makes the wire resistant to kinking. As the body is PTFE-coated there is no worry that the wire may slip out. The proximal end also has a flexible tip for retrograde passage of the flexible endoscope through the working channel without causing damage. Hybrid wires were designed to reduce the amount of time spent manipulating with different wires. Some argue they are a 'jack of all trades' and perhaps not a master of any. Some helpful hints on using guidewires are provided in Box 3.5.

TIP! **Hydrophilic wire**
- It is a very slippery wire. The commonest mistake of the inexperienced is either to pull the wire out inadvertently or to imagine they are inserting the wire, when in fact it is merely slipping through their fingers
- Easy in, easy out! One access established exchange for a standard PTFE wire as the hydrophilic wire may slip out
- Moisten regularly. A dry hydrophilic wire is less than useless. Use a saline-soaked swab before and during use to activate and maintain the hydrophilic coating

---

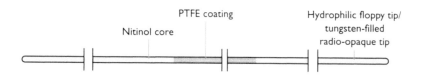

Figure 3.3 Illustration of the Sensor™ guidewire (courtesy of Boston Scientific).

Box 3.5 General tips on the use of guidewires

- Choose the correct wire for the task (see Table 3.2)
- Moisten well
- Keep the wire as straight as possible. Catheters are easier to insert over a straight wire
- Short jerks will succeed in advancing a catheter over a wire, when pushing does not
- Redundant loops should be avoided in the kidney or bladder
- Overpushing results in ureteral trauma
- With tight/total strictures gentle probing will succeed; undue force will not

Table 3.2 Wires and what they do

Wire type	Technical factors	Clinical use	Cost
PTFE	Low friction Teflon® coating	Cheap and should be first-line wire	+
Hydrophilic (Terumo)	Very slippery surface coating	Tortuous ureter; impacted calculi	+ +
Nitinol (Glidewire®)	Kink resistant Has memory	Good for difficult access	+ +
Hybrid wires (Sensor™)	Hydrophilic slippery tip; nitinol core resistant to kinking; flexible proximal tip	Fit for most difficult occasions	+ + +
Super stiff (Amplatz super stiff™)	Very kink resistant	Straightens out a tortuous ureter; used for dilatation of stricture or tracts for PCNL	+ +
Very floppy tip (Bentson)	Very safe, 8 or 15 cm floppy tips	Atraumatic tip; difficult to control in small spaces	+

Retrieval devices

An array of baskets and graspers are available for stone retrieval during ureterorenoscopy and percutaneous renal surgery. The device chosen is based upon stone and pathological factors, local anatomy and the type of equipment being used (flexible or rigid endoscopy). Personal experience and preference are equally as important.

Baskets and graspers vary in their opening mechanisms, and one must be aware of their action before passing the device into the scope. The device must always be checked to ensure it is intact before and after use. It can be a dangerous tool, with the potential to tear or detach the ureter if excess traction is applied. It must always be used with endoscopic/fluoroscopic control.

Baskets and their use

Basket devices are used to capture objects, calculi and stone fragments, and range in size from 1.9 to 7F. The average size is 3F in order to fit the working channel of most ureteroscopes. The device consists of a handle and a plastic sheath (Figure 3.4). Inside the sheath is a thin shaft of metal that forms the basket and a variety of basket shapes are available (Figure 3.5). The handle controls the opening of the basket. In the neutral state the basket is collapsed within the sheath. When the handle is turned, the basket comes out and expands. Some baskets open by withdrawal of the sheath. Detachable handles are available and are a necessary feature if the basket and stone becomes impacted during retrieval. Once detached from its handle, the endoscope can be withdrawn over the metal shaft leaving the stone and basket behind. The basket may then be dislodged from the stone by using intracorporeal lithotripsy with the ureteroscope passed alongside the basket wire.

Baskets may be made of stainless steel or nitinol. Nitinol has excellent shape memory, is much thinner and more elastic allowing greater miniaturisation of devices. This translates into greater irrigant flows and less impact on scope deflection during flexible ureterorenoscopy. The outer sheath is usually coated in PTFE. In certain baskets the sheath can be detached to reduce the overall size of the instrument in the working channel (bare-naked baskets) and improve the working ability of the flexible ureteroscope. Most baskets have a tip ranging from 1 to 9 cm in length beyond the basket. Hollow-core baskets have a central channel that allows for the passage of a guidewire or laser fibre.

All baskets have a minimum of three wires. The configuration of the basket design confers upon it specific retrieval characteristics (Table 3.3). Stone location (ureter vs intrarenal collecting system), multiplicity and size are important factors when selecting a basket.

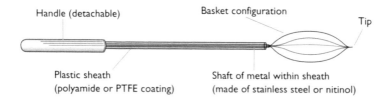

Figure 3.4 Standard design of a basket device.

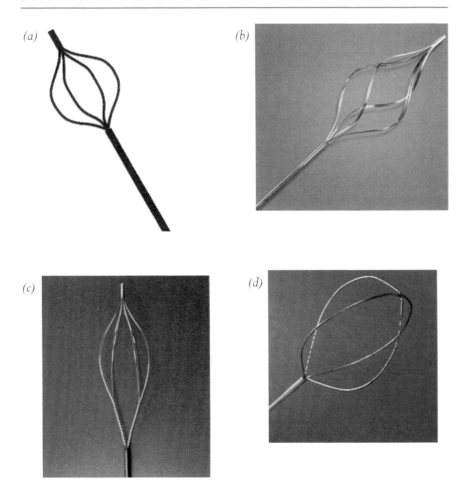

Figure 3.5 Different basket configurations.
(a) Flat-wire, (b) Helical (Gemini™ paired wire basket), *(c) Multiwire*
(Parachute™), *(d) Tipless* (ZeroTip™). *(Courtesy of Boston Scientific)*

Most basketing is successful and uncomplicated. Of problems, the mos
feared is the impacted basket after entrapment of the stone. The major limi
tation of current basket designs is that they are not designed to release
stone from the basket once captured. The common reason for an impacte
basket is that the basket with the captured stones will not pass through
narrow part of the ureter or stricture, e.g. the VUJ.

Table 3.3 Advantages and disadvantages of different basket designs

Basket configuration	Technical features	Advantages	Disadvantages
Flatwire (Segura™)	Consists of perpendicular loops of stainless steel flat wire; 2.4–4.5F	Easier stone capture Flat wires excise stalk of tumours Good for biopsy Good for large renal stones	Cause trauma to mucosa Difficult to disengage Not so good for multiple calculi Rarely used for URS
Helical (Dormia, Gemini™)	Up to 3 to 6 wires. Paired wires also available (Gemini™); 1.9–4.5F	Strong and easy to use Secure closure Can expand a narrow ureter Ideal for distal ureteric stones	Difficult to disengage stone Not good for smaller ureteral stones
Tipless (ZeroTip™)	Nitinol four-wire basket; 1.9–3F	Kink resistant Rapid stone extraction Less mucosal trauma Good release characteristics Ideal for calyceal stones	Expensive
Multiwire (Parachute™)	Eight-wire canopy; asymmetrical basket design, elongated to compress fragments into a long thin spindle facilitating extraction; 3F	Superior ability to retrieve multiple stone fragments Prevents proximal migration of calculus when opened above stone Like a net, smaller stones naturally fall into the centre of the basket	Does not occlude dilated ureters Bulky and can restrict the passage of other instruments in the ureter

Dretler stone cone

This is a nitinol device that consists of concentric coils (Figure 3.6). Although primarily designed to prevent retrograde migration of stone fragments during lithotripsy, it can also be used to retrieve stone fragments by capturing them within the coils as it is withdrawn distally.

Graspers

Like baskets, graspers are made from stainless steel or nitinol wires, encased in a sheath and controlled by a release handle. The three-pronged hooked grasper is the most widely used for ureteroscopy (its size varies from 1.9 to 5F) (Figure 3.7). The grasper is positioned close to the stone and the prongs are opened. To capture the stone, the prongs must be retracted back into the sheath. These devices do not hold the stone as securely as baskets but do allow easy disengagement from the stone if it becomes impacted and are therefore safer (Box 3.6).

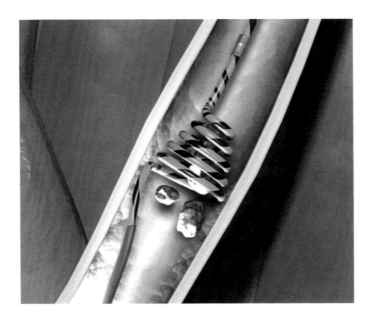

Figure 3.6 The Stone cone™. A nitinol coil that can prevent migration during stone fragmentation and sweep stone fragments in a single pass. (Picture courtesy of Boston Scientific)

(a)

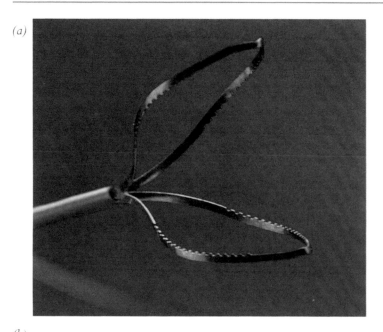

(b)

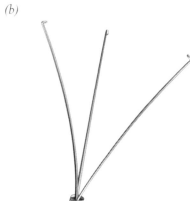

Figure 3.7 Flexible graspers and forceps used during ureterorenoscopy. (a) Nitinol retrieval forceps (2.6F or 3.2F). (b) Tri-radiate retrieval grasper (2.4 or 3.0F); the three-pronged hooked design allows for easy disengagement of the stone. (c) Intrarenal biopsy forceps (3F). (Pictures courtesy of Boston Scientific)

(c)

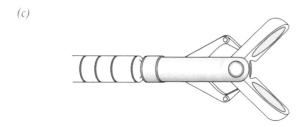

Box 3.6 Which one do I choose – basket or grasper?

Basket	Grasper
• Stone and basket can become impacted • Risk of ureteral wall trauma • Stone more secure	• Easy to disengage • Less trauma • Safer for retrieval in proximal ureter or calyces

---

Forceps

These simple reversible grasping devices have teeth for a better grip (alliga-tor or rat tooth). They are cheap, reusable and come in sizes ≥3F. Single-use flexible forceps are used during ureterorenoscopic stone extraction and for taking biopsies during semirigid ureteroscopy (cold-cup forceps) (Figure 3.7). Semirigid forceps of this nature are mostly used during percutaneous stone extraction (Figure 3.8).

Ureteral stents

Stents allow drainage of the urinary tract in the presence of obstruction from either intrinsic (e.g. calculi, strictures, blood clot, tumour, congenital abnor-malities) or extrinsic (e.g. retroperitoneal fibrosis, tumour) causes. When placed in the ureter they cause ureteric stasis. Urine flows both through and around the indwelling stent. In addition, stents allow 'structural scaffolding' by providing a bridge to promote healing and prevent stricture formation when the ureter is damaged or under repair. They can be inserted endo-scopically in a retrograde manner, percutaneously in antegrade fashion as well as placed at the time of open surgery.

Ureteral stents vary in their size, composition, design and surface coating. Box 3.7 lists the properties of the ideal stent. All present-day stents are a compromise to some degree. The perfect stent does not yet exist.

Size

The standard ureteral stent varies in its outer diameter from 4F to 8F and in length from 8 to 32 cm. Increasing the internal diameter of the stent

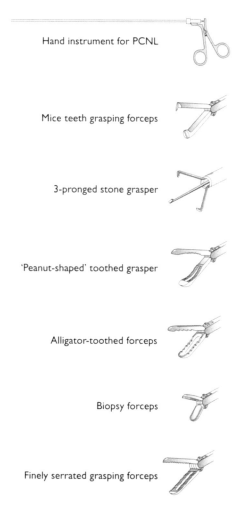

Hand instrument for PCNL

Mice teeth grasping forceps

3-pronged stone grasper

'Peanut-shaped' toothed grasper

Alligator-toothed forceps

Biopsy forceps

Finely serrated grasping forceps

Figure 3.8 Different forceps tip design available for percutaneous renal surgery. (Courtesy of Richard Wolf UK Ltd)

increases the urinary drainage, but at physiological flow rates, 5F to 8F ureteral stents show no major differences in pressure–flow characteristics. A 24 cm 7F ureteral stent is suitable for most adults. Sizing is important, as long stents will cause irritative bladder symptoms whilst short stents will migrate up the ureter. However, it should be remembered that manufacturers differ in how the stent length is measured – some use the tip-to-tip length, whilst others measure only the straight portion. Multilength stents are designed to fit all situations – their pigtails are made of multiple coils or turns and the pigtails unfurl and adjust to the length of ureter.

Box 3.7 The ideal stent

- Good memory (ability to maintain position within the ureter)
- Easily inserted and removed
- Good tensile strength to allow for a higher internal/external diameter ratio
- Greater number of side holes to improve urinary drainage
- Well tolerated with no significant effects on the urothelium (biocompatibility)
- Need to be durable (biodurability)
- Resist biofilm formation and infection
- Resist encrustation
- Resist migration
- Radio-opaque
- Low cost

Composition

Non-metallic stents

The earliest stents were made of polyethylene, silicone or polyurethane (Table 3.4). Modern stents are made from hybrid polymers, proprietary materials like C-flex® (Cook®), Percuflex® (Boston Scientific Urological Inc., IN, USA) or Silitek, MA, USA (ACMI, MA, USA). Metallic salts are added to make them radio-opaque to aid insertion or removal and monitor follow-up. Changes to the cross-linking used in these polymers can affect the strength of the material. Harder stents are more suited for urinary obstruction due to extrinsic compression from tumour while softer stents are said to be less irritative.

All stents develop a biofilm on insertion that consists of electrolytes, proteins, urea and microbes, eventually leading to encrustation, stent failure or infection. Whether prophylactic antibiotic administration during stent insertion has any impact upon biofilm formation is unclear.

In the future, bioabsorbable or autologous tissue engineered ureteric stents may be available. Bioabsorbable stents would maintain their structural features for a defined period, after which they would biodegrade *in situ*. This stent would obviate the need for stent removal and avoid the morbidity associated with forgotten stents (Box 3.8). Early results from *in vitro* and *in vivo*

Table 3.4 Ureteric stents

Material	Strengths	Weaknesses
Silicone	Resistant to encrustation Good biocompatibility	Low tensile strength High coefficient of friction
Polyurethane	Versatile Low friction coefficient High tensile strength	Poor biocompatibility (urothelial ulceration and erosion)
Polyethylene	Good biocompatibility	Encrustation Infection Poor biodurability
Silicone modified polymer (C flex®)	Good biocompatibility High retaining capacity	Encrustation
Polyester copolymer (Silitek®)	High tensile strength Good biodurability	High friction coefficient Encrustation
Olefinicblock copolymer (Percuflex®)	Good memory High durometry Low friction coefficient	Encrustation

Box 3.8 Stent durability

- All currently available plastic stents have a limited indwelling life (4–6 months depending on make of stent)
- All patients with stents should be maintained on regular follow-up and stents should be exchanged regularly
- The 'forgotten' stent can lead to substantial morbidity

studies have been promising (Lumiaho et al., 2000). The advantages of an autologous tissue stent are superior biocompatibility that eliminates encrustation.

All manufacturers claim improved resistance to encrustation with each new stent design. *In vitro* studies inform us about the benefits of some materials over others but present day technology has not yet resulted in a fully encrustation-free stent.

Metallic stents

Metallic stents have been effective in relieving urinary obstruction but are beset with problems of biocompatibility. Conventional metallic stents (e.g. the Wallstent®) are highly prone to re-stenosis as the urothelium grows through the stent interstices and gaps and most will seldom last more than a year before becoming blocked. More recently a nickel/titanium alloy stent (Memokath 051, Engineers and Doctors, Copenhagen, Denmark) has been developed that is biocompatible, thermo-expandable, good at maintaining its shape and, uniquely for metallic stents, easily removable. The Memokath stent can be left indwelling for a much longer period (up to 5 years in some cases) and is well tolerated by patients because it lacks retention coils in the kidney and bladder (Figure 3.9). Worldwide experience of these stents is limited, but they are proving to be useful in the palliative treatment of malignant ureteral obstruction (Kulkarni & Bellamy, 2001).

Surface coating

A hydrophilic coating on both the outer and luminal surface reduces the coefficient of friction and makes it easier for the stent to pass up the ureter or through a guidewire or stricture. The hydrogel coating has good biocompatibility, is less resistant to encrustation and does not induce as much ureteral irritation compared to older stents. There are, however, concerns about the length of time the coating is effective and encrustation will still occur if left *in situ* for prolonged periods.

Special stent designs

Coil: Stents have a retention coil on one or both of the tips to prevent migration (Figure 3.10). The original retention feature, a double J design, was an open-hook configuration. Now all stents possess a double-pigtail design, as they have a higher retention strength than the J design. Stents with only a single coil are used in urinary diversions.

Sutures: Some stents have a nylon suture attached to the distal end which can be left at the urethral meatus (Figure 3.10). This allows for stent removal without the need for a cystoscopy. However the thread can irritate the urethra and this method of removal is usually reserved for short-term insertion.

Side holes: Most stents have side holes along the whole length of the stent to improve urinary drainage, but some have holes only over the pigtails. There is no clear advantage of either type.

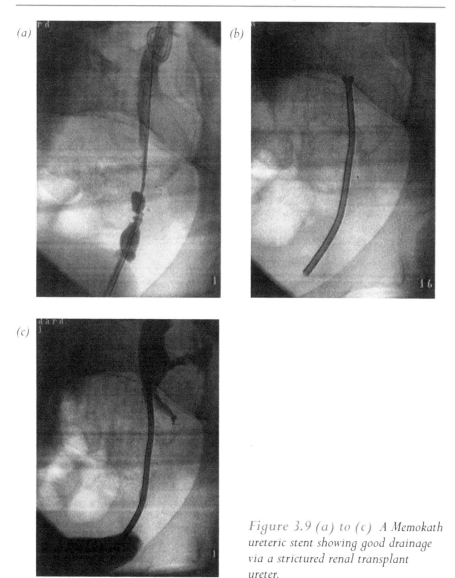

Figure 3.9 (a) to (c) A Memokath ureteric stent showing good drainage via a strictured renal transplant ureter.

Tail stents: This stent has a normal proximal portion (7F) whilst the distal segment is soft, narrow (3F), lumenless and without a coil. They are said to result in fewer stent-related irritative voiding symptoms and reflux associated flank pain (Dunn et al.), but the evidence is not strong. In addition, they are contraindicated in the presence of ureteral trauma and can be awkward to position accurately.

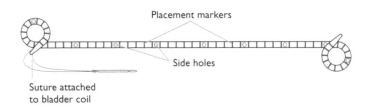

Placement markers

Side holes

Suture attached
to bladder coil

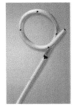

Figure 3.10 Typical pigtail ureteric stent with inset of atraumatic tapered insertion tip.

Endopyelotomy stents: This is a tapered stent, with a wider proximal portion suited for post-ureterotomy stenting (12–14F) and a narrower (6–7F) distal end. The thicker shaft is believed to provide a splint for ureteral healing while the narrower portion reduces stent-related symptoms.

Ureteral catheters

Ureteral catheters are open-ended tubes with no side holes. They have many varied functions and are used for most endourological procedures in the upper tract (Box 3.9). The olive-tipped catheter allows atraumatic insertion and the Chevassu/cone tip design is particularly useful for retrograde ureteric imaging. Dual lumen catheters can be used to insert both safety and working wires, or inject contrast or irrigation through the second lumen (Figure 3.11).

Box 3.9 Functions of a ureteral catheter

- Temporary urinary drainage
- Retrograde ureteropyelography
- Opacification of collecting system for percutaneous access
- Help gain access to ureteric orifice
- Exchange guidewires
- Obtain upper tract urine cytology and brushings
- Stiffen proximal wire for distal manipulations

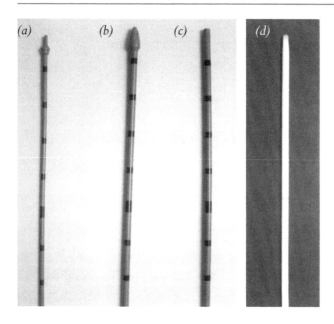

Figure 3.11
Ureteric catheters
(Boston Scientific).
(a) Wedge tip (4F),
(b) Cone tip (6F),
(c) Open ended (6F),
(d) Tapered tip (6F),
(e) Dual lumen
ureteric catheter

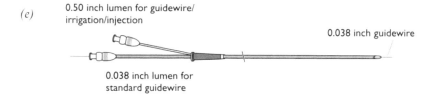

(e) 0.50 inch lumen for guidewire/ irrigation/injection

0.038 inch guidewire

0.038 inch lumen for standard guidewire

Ureteric access sheaths for flexible ureterorenoscopy

This sheath lies between the external urethral meatus and renal pelvis and allows repeated atraumatic passage of the flexible URS for lithotripsy and retrieval of stone fragments (Figure 3.12). They provide additional benefit in the form of a continuous flow of irrigant which improves vision and reduces intrarenal pressure. They are, however, relatively large with external diameters up to 12F and the trocar tips are still rather long, making access to the pelvi-ureteric junction (PUJ) difficult in small pelvicalyceal systems. In addition, some users consider post-operative stenting mandatory if an access sheath has been used due to full-length ureteric dilatation. The trend toward further miniaturisation of the endoscopes suggests that these excellent devices will become narrower and even less traumatic in time.

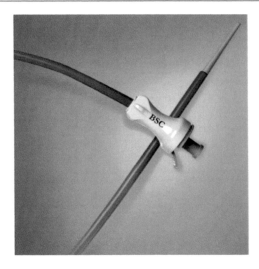

Figure 3.12 Ureteric access sheath. Tapered tip and hydrophilic coating allow relatively atraumatic insertion; removable trocar allows passage of flexi URS. (Courtesy of Boston Scientific)

Balloons and dilators

Box 3.10 What can you dilate?

- Intramural ureter and orifice
- Ureteric strictures
- Percutaneous tract
- Infundibular stenosis
- Calyceal diverticula

Balloon dilatation

Balloon dilators are quick, easy to use and relatively atraumatic. They are used extensively throughout medicine, particularly for radiologically guided intravascular work. In endourology, they may be used for upper tract endoscopy with inflation under vision for ureteric strictures, or inflation with contrast under fluoroscopic control (Box 3.10). The devices vary in balloon profile, compliance, shape, length and inflation pressures. The important features of a balloon are listed below. Tips on balloon dilatation are provided in Box 3.11.

Size: Length can vary from 2 to 12 cm and the outer diameter, when inflated, is between 4 and 10 mm (or 12–30F). For dilatation of ureteric strictures an 8 mm (24F) diameter is sufficient.

Compliance: This is the ability of the balloon to stretch. Ideal balloons are non-compliant, stretching minimally and equally along the entire length of the balloon with the same external diameter regardless of the extrinsic tissue to be dilated. When dilating ureteric strictures, non-compliant balloons should not develop an hourglass around the stricture.

Profile: This refers to the shape and the diameter of the balloon in its deflated position. Low profile balloons maintain the same outer diameter in the deflated state no matter how many times it has been inflated. This is an important feature for smooth passage through the ureter or working channel of the endoscope.

Strength: When inflated the balloon must be strong enough to withstand rupture. The balloon is inflated through a pressure gauge to pressures between 8 to 30 atm (Figure 3.13). Endourological work requires high pressure balloons.

Tip design: Longer tips help to negotiate tortuous anatomy.

Zero tip: These balloons have a flat end rather than a tapered end and thus allow full dilatation when limited space is available (i.e. calyceal diverticulum, calyx full of calculus).

Ureteral balloon catheters

The balloon is located at the distal end of the catheter. The catheter consists of two channels, a central one to allow the guidewire through, and the second for inflation of the balloon with dilute contrast material. Two radio-opaque markers indicate the balloon position. Most catheters are 65 to 75 cm long, but can be up to 150 cm. Transcystoscopic balloon catheters for intramural ureteric dilatation are 5F to 7F in diameter (Figure 3.14). Transureteroscopic balloon catheters are much smaller (3 to 3.8F). The Passport™ ureteric balloon dilatation catheter (Boston Scientific) is a guidewire (PTFE or hydrophilic coated) with a 3F balloon at its distal tip.

Box 3.11 Balloons – how to dilate a stricture or track

- Take note of the manufacturer's recommended inflation pressure – inflate gradually and never exceed the maximum!
- Gradual dilatation is better
- The balloon should be positioned so the tightest portion of the stricture is in the middle of the balloon
- The aim is to abolish the waist. The presence of mild extravasation is another excepted technical endpoint of success
- The duration and number of inflations required are a matter of dispute, and personal choice (an example is 1 minute duration repeated three times)
- Resistant strictures may require an Acucise balloon or a 'cutting' balloon

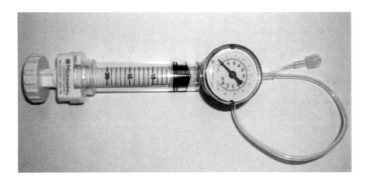

Figure 3.13 LeVeen inflation syringe. Luer lock connection and incorporated pressure gauge with screw mechanism for controlled balloon inflation. (Courtesy of Boston Scientific)

DO! Ensure all air is excluded from the system prior to balloon inflation.

Nephrostomy balloon dilators

Balloon catheters for percutaneous access allow one-step dilatation of the percutaneous tract under fluoroscopic monitoring. The expansive nature of the balloon exerts a lateral compressive force on tissues which is theoretically less traumatic than the shearing forces created with serial dilators. The

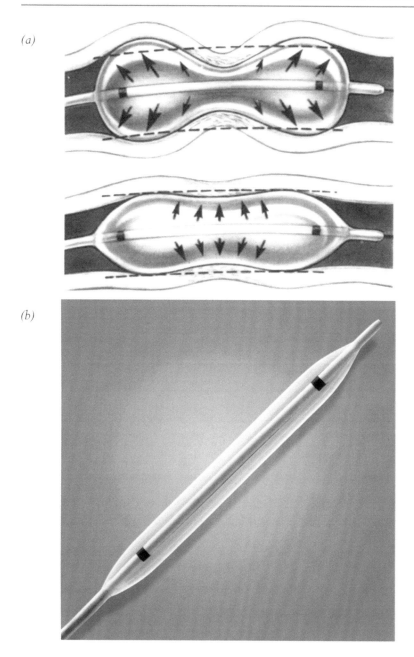

Figure 3.14 *Ureteric balloon dilatation. (a) A compliant balloon tends to hourglass around a stricture. In contrast, a non-compliant balloon retains its shape as it generates force against the stricture. (b) Ureteric balloon catheter. Radio-opaque markers indicate the length of the non-compliant balloon. (Courtesy of Boston Scientific)*

balloon which is on the tip of a 7F catheter is typically 12 cm in length and expands to 30F (approximately 10 mm). Once the tract has been created a 30F backloaded Amplatz working sheath is advanced over the catheter and the balloon deflated (Figure 3.15). Balloon dilatation is not as effective in the presence of dense scar tissue from previous surgery. Balloon dilators are considerably more expensive than re-usable metal dilators.

Presently zero tip balloons are not available for PCNL dilatation. Due to the graduated end, the dilatation must proceed for a centimetre or so to allow the Amplatz to reach the calyx. Therefore there must be room between the calyx and stone to accommodate the balloon. This is often not the case with staghorn calculi and stones in calyceal diverticula.

> **DO!** Before dilating, make sure the tip of balloon does not go beyond the calyx, as this may cause an infundibular tear

Solid dilators

Serial ureteral dilators

These flexible dilators can be used over a guidewire for cystoscopic or fluoroscopic dilatation of the ureteric orifice and intramural ureter. They are made of C-flex, Percuflex or polyethylene and range in size from 6F to 18F.

Percutaneous dilators

Many devices are available for tract dilatation and the method chosen is based upon patient factors, anatomy, personal experience and preference. All techniques require careful fluoroscopic monitoring during the procedure to prevent trauma to the pelvicalyceal wall.

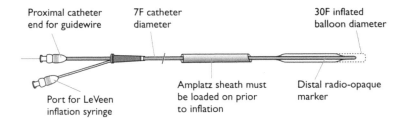

Figure 3.15 Balloon catheter for intrarenal access.

TIP! The final diameter of the tract should exceed the size of the instrument or drainage tube to be used by 2F.

Fascial dilators

These flexible catheter dilators can be used for a wide variety of interventional procedures. Starting with an 8F catheter that is fed over the guidewire, each catheter is replaced in a serial fashion by the next size up. This technique relies on careful guidewire control to prevent buckling in the collecting system. These dilators are quite flexible and not strong enough to overcome tough fibrous tissue.

Amplatz dilators

This set devised specifically for percutaneous access by Kurt Amplatz in the early 1980s improved on the fascial dilator design (Rusnak et al., 1982). Amplatz dilators are made of polyurethane, which makes them more rigid than fascial dilators, and able to dilate scar tissue. An 8F catheter is passed over the guidewire and kept in place to provide a catheter and guidewire combination over which progressively larger dilators (increments of 2F) are advanced (range 12–30F). After dilatation to the required size a thin-walled PTFE sheath (Amplatz sheath) is inserted over the dilator in a coaxial fashion and the dilator is removed (see Chapter 8).

Metal coaxial dilators

This set consists of a 58 cm long metal hollow rod that is passed over the guidewire (Alken or Lunderquist metal dilators). These dilators are re-usable. The tip of the rod is positioned within the collecting system and stainless steel concentric dilators are sequentially advanced over it (increasing in size by 4F). The telescopic dilators fit on top of each other tightly, with an interlocking edge that prevents progression beyond the tip of the rod. The potential for perforation of the renal pelvis is greater and considerable skill is required for this technique (Box 3.12). It is particularly suitable for patients with perirenal fibrous or scar tissue and, uniquely, it is a zero-tip dilatation system.

TIP! Metal dilators are very useful when wire access is precarious, for example when it is curled within a stone bearing calyx or diverticulum.

Box 3.12 Technique of dilatation with plastic or metal dilators

---

- Dilatation should be along the path of the wire or the wire will kink
- Dilatation is a combination of rotation and forward motion
- A 360° rotation is most effective
- Forward motion should be 1–2 cm at each 360°
- Forward motion/force should be released just before the end of each rotation
- Dorsiflexion at wrist and hyperextension of thumb helps during dilatation
- Progress in 4F steps – from 8F to 12F to 16F up to 24F. Take smaller steps (2F) if there is tough scar tissue

NON-DISPOSABLE EQUIPMENT

Intracorporeal lithotripsy

In the ureter, stones greater than 4 mm cannot be extracted whole and need to be fragmented to allow safe retrieval from the ureteric lumen. A range of lithotripsy devices are available (Figure 3.16) and the method chosen depends on various factors; these include the mechanism of action, suitability for rigid or flexible endoscopy, size, efficacy and safety considerations. The availability of equipment is usually dictated by the costs of hardware and disposable items.

Electrohydraulic lithotripsy (EHL)

This was the first intracorporeal lithotripsy device used. It is available for both rigid and flexible endoscopy. Stones are fragmented by shockwaves. An electrical spark is created which generates a cavitation bubble resulting in a shockwave that fractures the stone (Figure 3.16a). Energy from the cavitation bubble may spread beyond the target site and cause damage to the urothelium. As a result, there is a higher rate of ureteral trauma and perforation using EHL compared to other methods (Box 3.13).

(a)

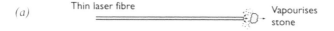

(b)

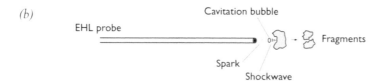

(c)

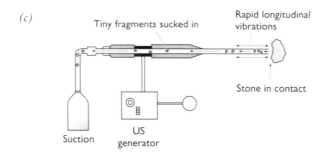

(d)

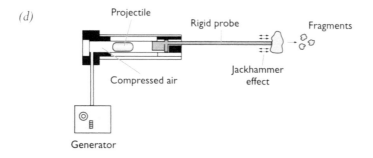

Figure 3.16 Mechanism of action of different intracorporeal lithotriptors.
(a) Laser, (b) EHL, (c) USL and (d) Pneumatic.

Ultrasound lithotripsy (USL)

Ultrasound lithotripsy was developed after EHL. Electrical excitation of a piezoceramic plate within the probe creates sound waves at frequencies of 23–27 kHz. These waves are transmitted to the tip and the resulting high frequency vibrations cause stone surface disintegration. Direct contact with the stone cuts a path through the stone by a drilling effect (Figure 3.16b).

Box 3.13 Tips on using EHL

- Ensure good saline irrigation
- Apply energy just proximal to stone surface
- Start on a rough surface
- Use a low energy charge and work way up
- Use short intermittent pulses
- Keep probe away from mucosa

Vibrations on the urothelium do not induce the same level of trauma as EHL. The probe generates heat and continuous irrigation is needed to prevent thermal injury. The fragments produced are very small and are aspirated through a hollow chamber in the probe (Box 3.14). However, the smaller 2.5F probe lacks this ability. A semiflexible 4.5F probe is available for URS, but is not as effective because the probe loses energy transmission when flexed. USL is less effective than EHL for very hard stones, e.g. oxalate stones.

Laser lithotripsy

Laser stands for *l*ight *a*mplification by *s*timulated *e*mission of *r*adiation. With laser a concentrated high energy beam of light is transmitted in the form of photons. Lasers are named after the laser medium generating the specific wavelength of light. They may be divided into continuous wave and pulsed wave types. Continuous wave lasers such as neodymium: ytrrium–aluminium–garnet (Nd:YAG) are not used for lithotripsy as they produce constant energy with undesirable thermal effects. These lasers are

---

Box 3.14 Tips on using USL

- Keep tip away from mucosa
- Keep probe in direct contact with stone
- Manipulate stone against wall with probe to ensure good contact
- Start working on a rough area of stone first
- Avoid taking out the middle of stone and leaving a difficult 'shell' to remove.
- Be patient!

---

more suited for ablative procedures (see Chapter 10). Pulsed wave lasers use pulsed energy resulting in little heat dissipation and very high power density at the stone surface.

> DO! Attendance on a laser safety course is compulsory before peforming laser lithotripsy

Pulsed-dye laser

Based on a coumarin dye system, this was the first widely used laser lithotriptor. Pulses (at 1 µs) of red light are emitted at a wavelength of 504 nm through optical quartz fibres (200–320 µm). Stone fragmentation occurs via a photo-acoustic effect. Laser light is absorbed by the stone leading to a plasma bubble on the surface which generates a shockwave. These machines are expensive to run and hard to maintain.

Holmium:YAG

This is the current standard for laser lithotripsy (Sofer et al., 2002). It is a compact and portable solid-state system and is widely used in other specialties (Figure 3.17). It is also a pulsed-wave laser, with a relatively long pulse duration (250 to 350 µs). The active medium is the rare earth element holmium with an yttrium–aluminium–garnet crystal. Light at a wavelength of 2150 nm is transmitted through small silica quartz fibres. The two main laser fibre sizes are 200 and 350 µm. All types of urinary calculi are vapourised into fine fragments and debris by a photothermal chemical effect (Box 3.15).

Pneumatic lithotripsy

Also known as ballistic lithotripsy, this works by using bursts of compressed air to fire a metal projectile within the handpiece onto a metal rod, which moves in a longitudinal manner like a jackhammer (Swiss Lithoclast®, Electromedical Systems, USA) (Figure 3.16d). The tip of the probe needs to be in contact with the stone. Fragmentation is independent of stone composition (Box 3.16). The mechanical action of the probe can be combined with integrated suction of fluid and debris. A flexible (nitinol) probe is available, although it is not as effective as the rigid probe as power is lost on deflection.

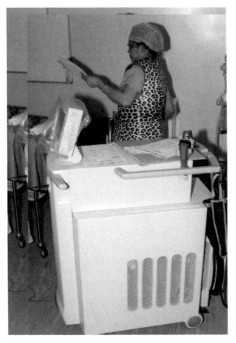

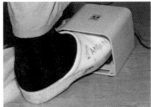

Figure 3.17 Holmium laser activated by footpedal with protective cover to prevent inadvertent laser firing.

Box 3.15 Tips on using holmium laser lithotripsy

- Ensure tip is out of the end of the scope before firing
- Ensure that aiming beam can be seen at all times
- Ensure flexible scope is straight before passing fibre to end of scope
- Do not laser the wire of baskets
- Keep at least 2 mm away from mucosa
- Use the 200 μm fibre if using with flexible scope and deflection
- Fragmentation is slow – be patient!

Box 3.16 Tips on using pneumatic lithotripsy

- Ensure direct vision of stone and probe
- Press stone gently against urothelium if migration is a problem
- Start with single pulse which can be very effective
- Fire several salvos at the same spot in the stone
- Keep attacking where a hairline break appears
- Fragment to sizes <3 mm

Combined US and Pneumatic lithotripsy

The Swiss Lithoclast Master® (Electromedical Systems, USA) is a relatively new lithotrite that combines a pneumatic probe within the hollow section of an ultrasound probe (Figure 3.18). Suction is maintained through the ultrasound probe. Both components are connected to a single control unit and may be used in combination or can be activated separately. *In vitro* studies have shown that combination lithotripsy is significantly more efficient than either modality on its own, particularly for large volume renal calculi (Auge et al., 2002).

Endoscopes

Over the last two decades advances in fibreoptics technology, miniaturisation of instrumentation and improvements in video imaging have led to both rigid and flexible upper tract endoscopy becoming standard procedures in urology departments the world over. All endoscopes have a standard design, consisting of a port for light transmission, an eyepiece for direct vision, one or two working channels for instrumentation and ports for irrigation if using a rigid endoscope.

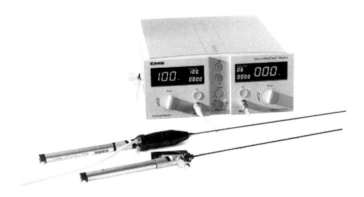

Figure 3.18 The Swiss Lithoclast Master® combines pneumatic and ultrasound lithotripsy in a single probe with simultaneous suction. (Courtesy of Electro Medical Systems)

Ureteroscopes

Endoscopic exploration of the upper urinary tract was first performed by Hampton Young in 1912 who inserted a cystoscope into the dilated ureter of a child. After that it was not until 1977 that Goodman published the first report of rigid ureteroscopy. Ironically, transurethral flexible ureteroscopy was performed a decade earlier by McGovern and Walzack (Marshall, 1964). Convenient ureteroscopy was only possible after Hopkins invented the rod-lens system for light transmission in endoscopes. Compared to the thin lenses of the past, the system of long rod-shaped glass cylinders interposed with air pockets devised by Hopkins increased the amount of light transmitted through smaller diameter endoscopes.

Rigid / semirigid ureteroscopy

First-generation rigid ureteroscopes were 13–16F (with a sheath) and did not have a working channel. Second-generation ureteroscopes were smaller (8.5–11F) and had a 3.5F working channel. These instruments were still fairly large and routine ureteral dilatation for access was the norm. Third-generation ureteroscopes used fibreoptic technology for light transmission which allowed them to be smaller (7.2F) with space for more than one working channel (2 × 2.1F). Unlike their predecessors, they could undergo gentle deflection without deterioration in vision, and came to be known as the semirigid ureteroscope. Following this, the mini-semirigid ureteroscope (6.9F) was introduced which had larger working channels (2.3F and 3.4F) (see Chapter 1, Figures 1.3–1.5).

With the modern semirigid ureteroscope, the need for ureteric dilation has been virtually abandoned. Semirigid ureteroscopy is routinely used for access to the distal and mid ureter, and sometimes to the proximal ureter and renal pelvis in women. A range of ureteroscopes is available from different manufacturers. Whilst most will have two working channels, slightly smaller ureteroscopes are available with only one working channel. An angled eyepiece design is also available to provide a straight working channel for rigid lithotripsy. The tip is bevelled to be atraumatic on the mucosa. As the shaft progresses proximally, it gradually gets larger in order to give the ureteroscope strength and stability.

Flexible ureterorenoscope

The flexible ureterorenoscope (flexi URS) provides access to the proximal ureter and intrarenal collecting system (see Chapter 1, Figure 1.4). Despite its tiny nature, modern flexible ureterorenoscopy provides good visualisation at a magnification of 30–50 times. Deflection at the tip of the scope is an important feature that permits access to the calyces. The addition of a single working channel allows irrigation and instrumentation. Over the years, miniaturisation of stone retrieval devices and the suitability of the holmium laser fibre have improved the efficacy of flexible URS, such that it is now the first line intervention for <1 cm lower pole calyceal stones.

Modern flexi URSs are differentiated by their size, deflection mechanism, degree of deflection and size of the working channel. Table 3.5 lists differences between semirigid and flexible endoscopes.

Deflection

Deflection at the tip may be either active (controlled by a lever) or passive. As the average angle between the upper ureter and the lower pole is around 140°, the standard active deflection range of 120–160° is usually sufficient to get into the lower pole. Recently, a flexi URS has been developed that has an active deflection of 270° in each direction (Karl Storz Endoscopy, Germany). Most flexi URSs have an active deflection point close to the tip

Table 3.5 Features of semirigid and flexible ureteroscopes compared

	Semirigid	Flexi URS
Size (length)	30–45 cm	54–70 cm
Size (diameter at tip)	4.5–11.9F 6.9F commonly used	4.9–11F 7.5F commonly used
Field of view	65–90°	60–90°
Angle of view	5–10°, telescopic lens	0–9° (most 0), limited depth of field
Eyepiece	Can have offset Allows rigid instrumentation	No offset
Working channel	1 or 2	1
Lithotripsy	US, Pneumatic, laser	EHL, Laser

(primary active deflection) and a passive deflection point proximal to this (secondary passive deflection) (Figure 3.19). This set up allows access to the entire intrarenal collecting system in up to 95% of patients. Dual active deflection ureteroscopes have an active secondary deflection mechanism controlled through a second lever instead of a passive mechanism. This flexi URS can get 360° downward flexion.

Working channel

The standard size of the working channel is 3.6F. Instruments must be passed through the working channel with the flexi URS in the neutral position to prevent damage at the deflecting segment. When instrumentation is in the working channel, deflection at the tip is limited.

Irrigation

As irrigation and instrumentation use only the single working channel available, poor irrigant flow is a problem during flexi URS. This can be overcome by using smaller instruments (<3F) and by using pressurised irrigation devices or forcefully injecting fluid through a hand-held or foot pedal syringe.

Durability

These delicate endoscopes have a much shorter life span than their semirigid counterparts. The average number of times a single flexi URS can be used without requiring repair is 30–40. The commonest fault is deterioration in

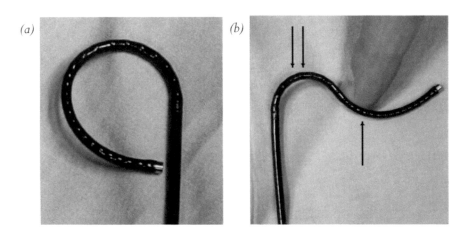

(a) (b)

Figure 3.19 Tip deflection of flexible ureterorenoscope; (a) shows a scope with 270° primary active deflection, (b) demonstrates the principles of primary active deflection (arrow) and secondary passive deflection (double arrows).

the deflecting mechanism of the tip. Nitinol instruments, smaller laser fibres (200 μm) and ureteral access sheaths can increase the longevity of flexi URS (Pietrow et al., 2002).

Nephroscope

Nephroscopy at open surgery was performed in 1972 with a dedicated right angle nephroscope (Vatz et al, 1972). With the advent of PCNL in the late 1970s, the role and value of nephroscopy suddenly increased. The rigid nephroscope is the workhorse instrument for PCNL. The standard adult nephroscope is made of stainless steel and is 24–26F in diameter (with sheath) (Figure 3.20). They are up to 21 cm in length with a single large working channel (13.5F). Flexible nephroscopes are similar to flexible ureteroscopes, but much shorter and larger (15F with 7.5F working channel).

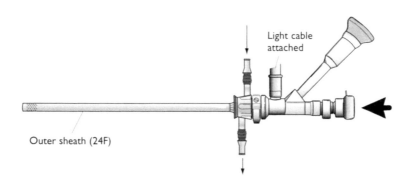

Light cable attached

Outer sheath (24F)

Figure 3.20 Standard design of rigid nephroscope. The scope illustrated here is fitted with its sheath, allowing continuous flow irrigation (arrows). Most people, however, use the scope without a sheath and have continuous irrigation around the scope within the Amplatz sheath. The eyepiece has an angled offset so that rigid instruments can be delivered into the 13.5F working channel (arrow head).

REFERENCES

Auge BK, Lallas CD, Pietrow PK, et al. In vitro comparison of standard ultrasound and pneumatic lithotrites with a new combination intracorporeal lithotripsy device. Urology 2002; 60: 28–32

Dunn MD, Portis AJ, Kahn SA, et al. Clinical effectiveness of new stent design: randomized single-blind comparison of tail and double-pigtail stents. J Endourol 2000; 14: 195–202

Goodman TM. Ureteroscopy with pediatric cystoscope in adults. Urology 1977; 9: 394

Kulkarni R, Bellamy E. Nickel–titanium shape memory alloy Memokath 051 ureteral stent for managing long-term ureteral obstruction: 4-year experience. J Urol 2001; 166: 1750–4

Lumiaho J, Heino A, Pietilainen T, et al. The morphological, in situ effects of a self-reinforced bioabsorbable polylactide (SR-PLA 96) ureteric stent; an experimental study. J Urol 2000; 164: 1360–3

Mashall VF. Fiber optics in urology. J Urol 1964; 110–4

Pietrow PK, Auge BK, Delvecchio FC, et al. Techniques to maximize flexible ureteroscope longevity. Urology 2002; 60: 784–8

Rusnak B, Castaneda-Zuniga W, Kotula F, et al. An improved dilator system for percutaneous nephrostomies. Radiology 1982; 144: 174

Sofer M, Watterson JD, Wollin TA, et al. Holmium: YAG laser lithotripsy for upper urinary tract calculi in 598 patients. J Urol 2002; 167: 31–4

Vatz A, Berci G, Shore JM, et al. Operative nephroscopy. J Urol 1972; 107: 355–7

SUGGESTED FURTHER READING

Elkabir J, Anson KM. Energy sources in urology. In Mundy AR, Neal D, George NJR, Fitzpatrick J, eds. Scientific Basis of Urology, 2nd edn. London: Martin Dunitz, 2004

4. Ureterorenoscopy

In this chapter we will address the anatomy relevant to ureterorenoscopy, consider the endoscopes available and describe the technique for diagnostic endoscopy including some tricks of the trade. Specific therapeutic interventions will be described in each relevant clinical chapter.

SEMIRIGID URETEROSCOPY

Ureteric anatomy

The adult ureter is approximately 22–30 cm long, varying in direct relation to the height of the individual. It follows a gentle sinusoidal curve from the pelviureteric junction (PUJ) to the vesicoureteric junction (VUJ). In the normal state the urine is transported from the renal pelvis via the ureter to the bladder by the peristaltic action of the ureteric muscle. The ureter receives its blood supply from multiple feeding arterial branches from the renal artery, or directly from the aorta or the superior vesical artery.

Box 4.1 Three things to know about the ureter

- 3 mm in diameter (standard)
- 3 layers: outer fibrous coat, middle muscular coat, inner mucous coat
- 3 relative areas of narrowing: at the pelviureteric junction, where the ureter crosses the iliac vessels and where it travels through the bladder wall

---

The ureter is covered by posterior peritoneum and the juxtavesical portions are embedded in vascular retroperitoneal fat (Box 4.1). From the renal pelvis it travels inferiorly on the psoas muscle and then enters the lesser pelvis by crossing anterior to the iliac vessels (Figure 4.1). It then descends posterolaterally on the lateral wall of the pelvis. Just opposite the ischial spine, it turns anteromedially to run above the levator ani and then enters the

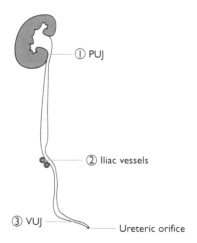

Figure 4.1 The ureter has three relative areas of narrowing.

base of the bladder. In both sexes the ureter enters the bladder posterolaterally and courses submucosally to enter the bladder at the ureteric orifice. The orifices are generally found 1 to 2 cm proximal to the bladder neck and are bridged by a ureteric bar and normally face medially, forming an oblique slit. The cystoscopic appearances of the orifices are altered by the degree of bladder distension. In complete ureteric duplication the origins of each ureter can be difficult to visualise. The VUJ and the intramural ureter are the narrowest segments of the ureter and intubation of these areas is often the most challenging part of diagnostic ureteroscopy. The ureter is rather arbitrarily divided into segments for surgical and imaging descriptions (Box 4.2).

Box 4.2 The three segments of the ureter

(1) Upper ureter: extends from the PUJ to the upper border of the sacrum
(2) Middle ureter: between the upper and lower border of the sacrum
(3) Lower ureter: extends from the lower border of the sacrum to the bladder

---

Semirigid ureteroscopes

Rigid ureteroscopy became a routine procedure in the late 1970s and early 1980s. The initial ureteroscopes were 13–16F in diameter and were based on traditional cystoscope design with interchangeable telescopes. However, they were difficult to deliver into the ureter and over time the endoscopes have become smaller and more flexible, and have vastly improved optics.

Modern day ureteroscopes are considered semirigid due to the thin, gently malleable metal sheath. They incorporate fibre optic bundles for image and light transmission and have working channels of up to 5.5F. The most recent advance has been in the design of two separate working channels to allow so-called continuous flow irrigation and to allow the use of two completely separate ancillary instruments simultaneously. Traditionally the ureteroscopes were manufactured with a narrow tip and a gradually widening shaft toward the eyepiece (see Chapter 1, Figure 1.3).

This design provides the necessary rigidity to the endoscope, however the larger proximal diameter can prevent passage of the endoscope further up the ureter. With modern materials the most recent endoscopes have sufficient strength whilst retaining a constant narrow diameter from tip to proximal shaft. They are, however, increasingly malleable as a result and may bend during the procedure. They can be manually straightened after the procedure with some care!

TECHNIQUE OF URETEROSCOPY

Ureteroscopy is one of the core skills of the endourologist and requires a working knowledge of the individual patient anatomy, endoscope design and ancillary instruments available. Like most endoscopy, it is easy when it is easy but when it is difficult, it can prove to be extremely difficult. The aim of all ureteroscopy is to provide the diagnostic and therapeutic intervention with as little morbidity as possible. Recently the routine use of post-operative ureteric stenting after ureteroscopy has been called into question and in our experience stenting is the exception rather than the rule. Whilst this is a great advance for the patient it does require increased levels of skill for the endoscopist. Extra care should be taken at all stages to reduce the risk of post-operative ureteric obstruction from blood, oedema, retained stone fragments, etc.

Pre-procedure assessment and patient positioning

Before the operation the surgeon should review the indications for ureter-oscopy and confirm the side of the procedure with the patient and with the most up to date imaging. All the necessary instruments should be available and the image intensifier and radiographer should be in theatre. Care should be taken with patient and instrument positioning. The patient should be positioned in a satisfactory position on a radiograph-compatible table with fluoroscopic access up to the top of the kidney. The patient position should provide the easiest access to the penis (in the male), bladder and full length of the ureter. In our experience the Lloyd-Davies position is the most valuable, as it enables the surgeon to manipulate the legs intraoperatively (Figure 4.2).

DO! The arms of the patient should be extended along the patient's body with the hands secured to the trunk to keep them out of the way during fluoroscopy

---

The video monitor and image intensifier should be in the surgeon's most comfortable line of sight to reduce the need to bend or rotate the neck (Figure 4.3). Roof-mounted combined monitors are ideal (Figure 4.4). The endoscopist needs to be able to sit as comfortably as possible, and for prolonged procedures an 'armchair' with back and arm rests can be invaluable. The theatre environment is hugely important; the surgeon needs to be as comfortable and relaxed as possible with minimal outside distractions in order to concentrate on the task at hand.

Ureteroscopy

The procedure starts with standard cystourethroscopy to define the urethral, prostatic and bladder anatomy. Most attention should be paid to the number and position of the ureteric orifices. The larger field view offered by the cystoscope is valuable in identifying these landmarks, as finding awkward ureteric orifices with the narrow view of the ureteroscope can prove very frustrating (Box 4.3).

(a)

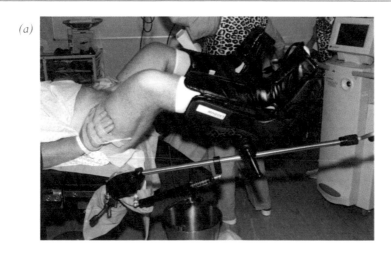

(b)

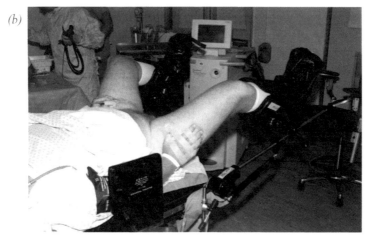

Figure 4.2(a) and (b) The Lloyd-Davies position for upper tract endoscopy. Note the adjustable leg supports, patient's bottom at the end of the table and hands taped to the side.

DO! If the orifices are considered 'difficult' at cystoscopy then place a guidewire into the ureter via the cystoscope to aid ureteroscopic localisation

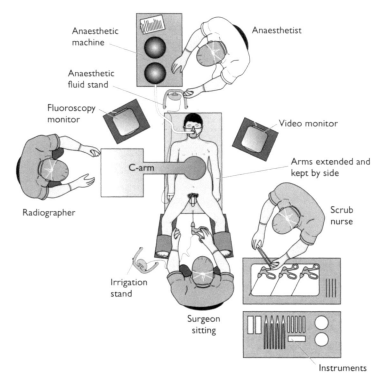

Figure 4.3 Theatre set-up for ureterorenoscopy (configuration for left URS is shown). Positions of C-arm and monitors are reversed for right URS.

If the ureteric orifices remain elusive a number of other aides can be utilised (see Table 4.1 and Box 4.4). In abnormal positions, patience and gentle endoscopy with minimal trauma to the tissues are the secret to success. At the end of the cystoscopy it is sensible to leave the bladder empty.

Passing a guidewire into the ureter

A wire may be used for all ureteroscopies by some surgeons and others may only ever use them in difficult cases. Either way, the insertion of the wire must be performed safely. Using a rigid cystoscope a standard 0.038 inch straight-ended floppy-tip wire is passed through the instrument channel of a catheterising element incorporating an Albarran deflecting bridge.

The wire is confirmed to be in the correct position within the channel and under the deflecting bridge. The cystoscope is rotated toward the ureteric orifice and the wire passed into the middle of the lumen of the orifice and gently advanced under fluoroscopic control and looped in the kidney. If

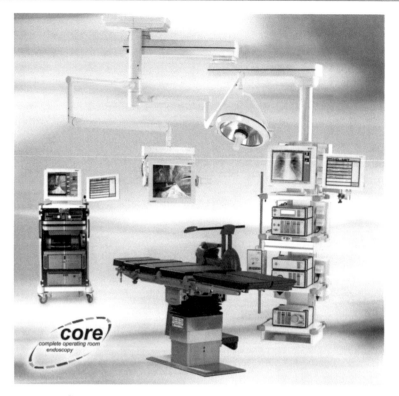

Figure 4.4 *Roof-mounted monitors and all other theatre equipment are centrally controlled, freeing up floor space, as demonstrated in this state of the art Wolf Complete Operating Room Endoscopy (CORE). (Courtesy of Richard Wolf UK Ltd)*

resistance is felt the procedure is stopped and the wire withdrawn. A further attempt is then made and this is often successful. The guidewire can then be referrred to as either a working or safety wire depending on its subsequent role and Box 4.5 and Figure 4.5 illustrate the differences in terminology.

DO! Position the cystoscope in the middle of the bladder so that inadvertent injury to the ureteric orifice does not occur as the wire emerges into view

DO! If a guidewire cannot be advanced, place an open-ended ureteric catheter over the wire which is then withdrawn, and perform a retrograde ureterogram to define the distal anatomy and exclude space-occupying lesions impeding passage

---

Box 4.3 Step-by-step guide to localise the ureteric orifices

(1) Empty the bladder
(2) Position endoscope at bladder neck
(3) Put on gentle irrigation to distend the bladder slowly and to open the orifice when viewing it end on
(4) Move forward very slowly and look downward
(5) Locate interureteric bar as thick band of muscle running transversely at the base of the trigone
(6) Gently move the endoscope along the interureteric bar and the ipsilateral orifice should be located on the inferior aspect of the interureteric bar at approximately 30° to the midline
(7) The contralateral orifice is then located by repeating this movement along the interureteric bar in the opposite direction (this manoeuvre can be employed to locate a ureteric orifice by finding the opposite one first)

Box 4.4 Still can't find the orifice and access is mandatory? Consider:

(1) Parenteral methylene blue/diuretics
(2) Percutaneous nephrostomy and antegrade stent placement. Come back another day and use a stent to guide you into the orifice
(3) Rendezvous procedure involving synchronous combined antegrade and retrograde manipulations to cross an impassable ureteric stricture

---

If the anatomy is normal but awkward a hydrophilic wire can be used and this will often pass. If still difficult, the cystoscope can be advanced right up to the ureteric orifice to offer some rigidity or a ureteric catheter can be passed over the wire for similar reasons. If success is still elusive, then an attempt with direct vision ureteroscopy may be successful and a wire passed via the ureteroscope with fluoroscopic control. However, direct vision ureteroscopy requires some experience and should not be attempted without care.

If the orifice still cannot be intubated by either the ureteroscope or guidewire then the procedure should be abandoned, and a percutaneous nephrostomy considered if appropriate. Further attempts at endoscopic

Table 4.1 Access to the difficult ureteric orifice

In normal position	In abnormal positions
(1) Change the amount of fluid in the bladder to alter the orientation of the orifice to the endoscopist	(1) Ectopic ureteric orifices can be found above and lateral to the normal orifice and anywhere along the trigone, and even down into the membranous urethra
(2) Gently caress the interureteric bar with a soft-tipped guidewire and often the wire will fall into the orifice 'blindly'	(2) Re-implanted orifices typically lie laterally and superiorly to the trigone. The neocystostomy of the transplant ureter is often easy to find, but difficult to intubate and endoscope
(3) Use downward deflection of the catheter bridge to apply some gentle pressure to the wire to explore the area	(3) After TURP, when the trigone has been encroached upon, the orifices may be very close to the bladder neck and can be very difficult to locate
(4) Check the top of the interureteric bar for awkwardly angled, normally positioned orifices	(4) After TURBT involving the orifices they may be wide open and refluxing, and quite lateral in position. Occasionally the opposite can occur if excess fulguration was used and then the orifice may be scarred and extremely narrow and elusive
(5) Change the cystoscope lens to 70° or 120° lenses	(5) Ileal conduit and bladder reconstructions: an understanding of the original operation is vital with particular attention paid to where and how the ureters were anastomosed. Often the orifices will fall into view and may appear as areas of normal looking urothelium surrounded by intestinal mucosa
(6) Use flexible cystoscope for awkward situations if above does not work (such as large middle lobe of the prostate)	

intervention should be delayed for a few days or more to allow the inevitable iatrogenic oedema to settle down. Once the wire has been successfully placed in the kidney the bladder should be emptied and the wire secured to the drapes, with care taken not to kink it.

> ## Box 4.5 Guidewire, safety wire or working wire?
>
> As they come out of the packet all wires are called guidewires. They adopt the names below once in use:
>
> *Safety wire*: if URS proceeds alongside the wire, the wire is acting as a safety wire and should be called that during the procedure
>
> *Working wire*: when manipulations are performed over a wire, such as passage of ureteric catheter, dilators or balloon, it is called a working wire

Intubation of the ureteric orifice

Once the bladder is emptied the position of the wire in the kidney is monitored fluoroscopically as the cystoscope is removed. The surgeon then stands to prepare and lubricate the ureteroscope, which is passed via the centre of the lumen of the urethra and prostate into the bladder. Once the bladder has been entered the surgeon can sit down comfortably. He or she must ensure all the ancillary equipment is in place before considering intubation of the ureteric orifices.

> DO! Keep an eye on the position of the tip of the ureteroscope at all times

In most situations the ureteroscope is passed alongside the safety wire, but some advocate an 'over the guidewire' technique whilst others will intubate with no wire in place. Once the ureteric orifice is located the ureteroscope is gently advanced through the ureteric lumen. Some gentle resistance is usually encountered at this stage, but after a short wait the ureter will open with peristalsis and the ureteroscope should only be passed further when the lumen is seen as open ahead of the endoscope. Once the intramural ureter has been negotiated the ureteroscope usually passes into a rather more dilated distal ureter and this is often accompanied by a slight give as the ureteroscope is advanced.

When intubation is easy the rest of the ureteroscopy can proceed as described below. However, often intubation is not straightforward and further techniques need to be employed (Box 4.6).

(a)

(b)

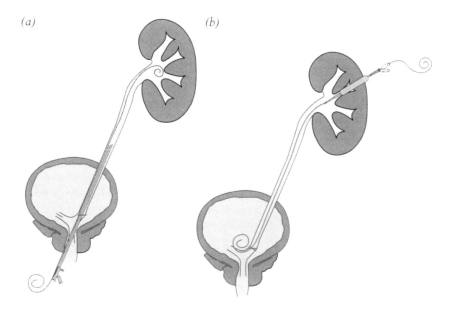

(c)

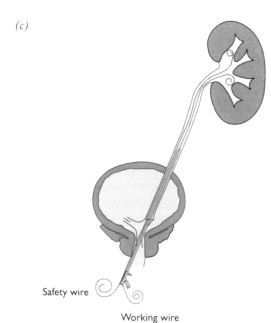

Safety wire

Working wire

Figure 4.5 Guidewire: safety wire or working wire? (a)Wire acting as a safety wire: ureteroscopy proceeds alongside the guidewire. (b)Wire acting as a working wire: in this case tract balloon dilatation. (c) Some prefer to use a safety wire alongside the working wire.

Box 4.6 Intubating the difficult ureter

---

(1) Dilate the ureter by increasing the hydrostatic pressure:

- Raise the height of the irrigant solution
- Squeeze the inflow tubing
- Use a syringe via the inflow tap

(2) 'Shoehorning': invert the ureteroscope to allow the bulky end of the ureteroscope to pass on the floor of the ureteric orifice (Figure 4.6). This can be particularly effective when using the 'over the wire' technique

(3) 'Riding the tracks': this can be mimicked in the safety wire technique by using a second wire through the ureteroscope. This wire is passed into the orifice and the ureteroscope rotated so that the two wires are aligned 180° to each other and the endoscope is then passed between the two wires (Figure 4.7)

(4) Dilatation of the ureteric orifice:

- Passive: over a few days with placement of a ureteric stent (requires a second procedure)
- Active: at the time with either serial ureteric dilators or balloon dilatation (can be performed either cystoscopically with fluoroscopy or by fluoroscopy alone)

Ureteroscopic navigation

Once the distal ureter has been entered the ureteroscope should be gradually advanced to the kidney using the principles of basic endoscopy outlined in Chapter 1 (Figure 4.8). Particular care should be taken not to push and to use 'soft hands'. As the endoscope advances through the middle of the lumen one should ensure that the ureteric wall moves in relation to the endoscope. If this is not occurring then the ureter is tight and being stretched, with the potential of serious consequences. In this case, the ureter could be further dilated, but perhaps common sense should prevail and the ureter stented and the procedure repeated at a later date. Often in this situation the ureter is more accommodating.

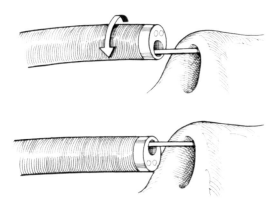

Figure 4.6 Shoehorning: by turning the instrument channel to the 12 o'clock position, the ureteroscope will not hit the roof of the ureteric orifice. Adapted from Figure 97.2. In Walsh PC, Retik AB, Vaughan ED Jr, et al., eds. Campbell's Urology, Vol. IV, 8th edn. Philadelphia: W.B. Saunders, 2002; with permission.

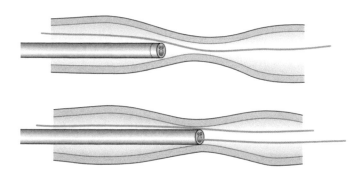

Figure 4.7 Riding the tracks: by using two wires as demonstrated, the narrowed segment of the ureter can be negotiated with the ureteroscope. Adapted from Figure 97.1 In Walsh PC, Retik AB, Vaughan ED Jr, et al., eds. Campbell's Urology, Vol. IV, 8th edn. Philadelphia: W.B. Saunders, 2002; with permission.

> **DO!** If performing active ureteric dilatation a ureteric stent should be placed post-operatively for at least one week

Certain areas of narrowing are encountered on the journey up the ureter. The iliac vessels at the pelvic brim often impede the passage of the endoscope. The ureter appears to travel at an almost impossible angle anteriorly

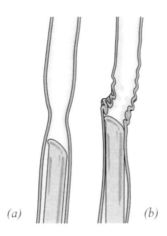

(a)   (b)

Figure. 4.8 Passage of ureteroscope. (a) The centre of the lumen should be visible at all times. (b) If not, the ureter may bunch and telescope on the ureteroscope.

Box 4.7 Getting past difficult points

(1) A wire can be passed via the endoscope to lie posteriorly in the ureter, thus pushing the ureter down and allowing the bulk of the scope to pass over the wire into the upper ureter (Figure 4.9)

(2) Fluoroscopic retrograde ureterogram via the instrument channel can identify the exact course of the ureter ahead

(3) A hand can be placed on the abdomen to push the ureter posteriorly and temporarily bring the full lumen into view

(4) The ureteroscope can be rotated, altering the orientation of the oval-shaped sheath within the lumen

(5) The two wire 'riding the tracks' technique (Figure 4.7) can be used

(6) A balloon can be passed via the ureteroscope to gently dilate the ureter under vision

---

and, despite manipulations, the lumen cannot be safely visualised. A number of techniques can be employed here and elsewhere in the ureter (Box 4.7).

Using a combination of these techniques the ureteroscope can usually be passed along the full length of the ureter or to the areas of interest. As long as care is taken and the procedure is performed calmly and steadily, and without undue force, it can be a most satisfying and enjoyable operation. If problems

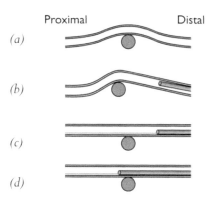

Figure 4.9 *Use of guidewire to ease passage of the ureteroscope over iliac vessels (lateral view). (a) Normal angulation of ureter over vessels; (b) ureteroscope lifted upward straightens distal ureter; (c) guidewire passed through ureteroscope straightens posterior wall of ureter; (d) ureteroscope passed over guidewire into proximal ureter.*

> TIP! Excellent views of the ureter are gained when removing the endo-scope and particular attention should be paid to whether a stone has been 'missed' as it is often possible to locate it on the way out.

are encountered anywhere along the journey and cannot be overcome it is much better to stent the ureter and come back another day rather than risk irreparable damage to the ureter and associated renal unit. Discretion is definitely the better part of valour when performing ureteroscopy.

FLEXIBLE URETERORENOSCOPY

Pelvicalyceal anatomy

The PUJ is often recognised at endoscopy by a narrowing of the upper ureter and a lateral ridge that appears to indent the ureter at this level. It alters con-figuration as the mobile renal pelvis moves caudally in relation to the rela-tively static upper ureter during inspiration. In contrast, during expiration the junction appears to elongate and can open.

> TIP! The optimum time for gaining retrograde endoscopic access to the renal pelvis is following a peristaltic contraction during expiration

The renal pelvis is then entered and this is recognised by a large, dark, capacious area with perhaps a few infundibulae in view. One can be confused at this point by either a bifid renal pelvis or a partial duplex ureter and a retrograde ureteropyelogram will provide the definitive answer if unsure. The pelvicalyceal region has a varied inter- and intrapersonal anatomy and needs to be fully appreciated in each renal unit for successful ureterorenoscopy. On average, the pelvicalyceal volume is 10–15 ml, but can be up to a few hundred ml in longstanding hydronephrosis. There are usually three renal calyceal groups – the upper, interpolar and lower pole calyces. The upper and lower calyces tend to be compound and project toward the polar region at various angles. The calyces drain via infundibulae into the renal pelvis. Generally the calyces are arranged in two rows that lie in the anterior and posterior plane (see Chapter 5 on percutaneous access). The kidneys lie on the psoas muscles with an approximate 30° anterior rotation to the coronal plane, and this brings the posterior lying calyces almost perpendicular with the overlying skin. In addition, the upper poles tilt slightly inwardly, as demonstrated in Figure 4.10. An appreciation of all of these anatomical details of the pelvicalyceal anatomy improves one's enjoyment and navigational success with flexible ureterorenoscopy.

Flexible ureterorenoscopes

The first flexible ureterorenoscopes were initially purely diagnostic, with no instrument channel and limited active deflection capabilities. In the late 1980s and early 1990s the modern generation of endoscopes were introduced with small atraumatic tips of 2–3 mm diameter, working channels up to 1 mm diameter and both active and passive deflection portions allowing up to 180° of deflection at the tip. As a result, both diagnostic and therapeutic ureterorenoscopy became a reality. Further refinements of these flexible endoscopes have provided superior image quality, slightly larger instrument channels and greater degrees of deflection (including in two separate planes), and all with greater durability. The capital costs and fragility of the endoscopes are a problem for all urology departments, but large centres treating many patients can justify the added expense. As fibreoptic technology develops, the improvements in design are likely to result in more durable and cheaper endoscopes that will be affordable for most departments. The next improvements that can be anticipated are videoureterorenoscopes with small CCDs at the tip and perhaps cheap, disposable, single-use instruments.

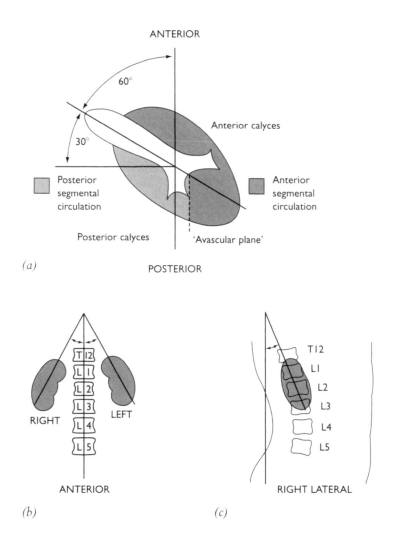

Figure 4.10 *Renal anatomy pertinent to ureterorenoscopy. (a) Transverse view showing approximate 30° anterior rotation of the left kidney from the coronal plane, relative positions of the anterior and posterior rows of calyces and location of the relatively avascular plane separating the anterior and posterior renal circulation. (b) Coronal section demonstrating slight inward tilt of the upper poles of the kidneys. (c) Sagittal view showing anterior displacement of the lower pole of the right kidney. Adapted from Figure 1.27. In Walsh PC, Retik AB, Vaughan ED Jr, et al., eds. Campbell's Urology, Vol. I, 8th edn. Philadelphia: W.B. Saunders, 2002; with permission.*

TECHNIQUE OF FLEXIBLE URETERORENOSCOPY

Many urologists will have already performed preliminary semirigid uretero-scopy (as outlined above) as a prelude to flexible ureterorenoscopy. This has two advantages, first excellent diagnostic views of the ureter are obtained and second it leads to some gentle dilatation of the ureteric orifice by the ureteroscope, thus aiding the passage of the flexible ureterorenoscope. A guidewire is left in the ureter with some contrast present within the pelvica-lyceal system. The flexible ureterorenoscope is placed over the guidewire.

> **DO!** Keep the endoscope light off initially to allow accurate placement of the wire in the instrument channel without scratching the image or light bundle

The wire is held firmly by an assistant (providing counter traction) and the endoscope is advanced over the wire, ensuring that it moves away from the assistant's hands holding the wire. The assistant will need to adjust their hand position on the wire as the scope advances. Combined fluoroscopic and endoscopic passage is ensured as the endoscope enters the ureter and passes gradually up and into the renal pelvis. The wire is then removed to allow full examination of the system. It is imperative that fluoroscopy is used at all times during passage to ensure that the wire is not inadvertently pulled into the endoscope at any stage by a rather overenthusiastic assistant, or even an overenthusiastic endoscopist!

With this approach no safety wire is kept in place for the procedure. An alternative, therefore, is to use a safety wire as well as a working wire, using a dual lumen catheter to place the two wires correctly as advocated by Kumar et al., 2001. A further approach is to pass the endoscope up through the lumen of a catheter that is positioned within the renal pelvis and outside the urethra, thus providing an easy conduit straight into the collecting system from outside the body (the 'access' sheaths). These vary in outer diameter from 11 to 15F and in length from 35 to 50 cm. They are particularly valu-able when performing prolonged interventions such as laser lithotripsy, where the combined convenience of easy retrieval of fragments and re-entry is possible and where the risks of rises in intrarenal pressures are best avoided (single kidney, recent urosepsis, etc.). In addition, the simultaneous drainage of the pelvicalyceal system during the endoscopy makes access sheaths useful when the view is suboptimal, but not when distension of the pelvicalyceal system is an advantage (the sheaths can be withdrawn below the PUJ in this situation). It is probably sensible always to leave a ureteric stent in place after using an access sheath due to their relatively large outer diameter. In contrast, for uncomplicated ureterorenoscopy post-operative drainage is not always required.

One important variation to the above protocol is for diagnostic ureterorenoscopy for small abnormalities (such as filling defects on IVU or upper tract haematuria). In this particular situation the guidewire should not be advanced beyond the extent of the rigid ureteroscopy navigation to prevent inadvertent trauma to the pelvicalyceal urothelium. This can mimic lesions and confuse the endoscopist. In addition, small amounts of bleeding can occur, thus obscuring views.

The pelvicalyceal roadmap

Once in the renal pelvis, systematic evaluation of the entire pelvicalyceal (PC) system should take place. In our institution this is aided by an assistant drawing a map of the entire pelvicalyceal system on the white board within theatre (Figure 4.11). The calyces are numbered sequentially from the superior aspect downwards and these can then be ticked off as they are inspected. In addition, further valuable reference information can be obtained by keeping the same retrograde image of the whole system on display on the second image intensifier screen throughout the procedure. It is surprising how easy it is to become disorientated and lost within the kidney and regular short flashes of fluoroscopy can be invaluable (if only to confirm that you are in the lower pole rather than the upper pole!). As for ureteroscopy, saline irrigation is used throughout and additional hydrostatic pressure can be applied as described above. Clearly care must be taken to prevent any significant rises in intrarenal pressure, but these techniques can be particularly valuable when irrigant flow becomes poor when an instrument is passed into the instrument channel. Specific techniques for intervention will be discussed in the relevant clinical chapter.

Once inspection has been completed the endoscope should be removed with care. As with ureteroscopy, excellent second-look views can be obtained when removing the instrument. The bladder should be emptied and then the patient can be woken up and taken to recovery.

DO! Consider a urethral catheter if:

- The procedure has been unduly long
- There has been bleeding throughout the procedure
- There is a concern about urosepsis
- The patient is an elderly man with an obstructing prostate

(a)

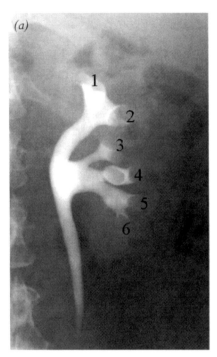

(b)

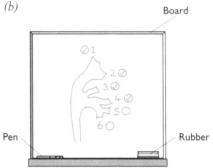

Figure 4.11 The 'road map'. The calyces are numbered as shown in (a). A schematic of the PC system is drawn on a board in theatre (b) with any noted abnormalities. As each calyx is entered, the assistant crosses it off on the schematic.

REFERENCES

Kumar PV, Keeley FX, Timoney AG. Safe flexible ureterorenoscopy with a dual-lumen access catheter and a safety guidewire. BJU Int 2001; 88: 638–9

SUGGESTED FURTHER READING

Bagley DH. Intrarenal access with the flexible ureteropyeloscope: effects of active and passive tip deflection. J Endourol 1993; 7: 221–4

Landman J, Monga M, El-Gabry EA, et al. Bare naked baskets: ureteroscope deflection and flow characteristics with intact and disassembled ureteroscopic nitinol stone baskets. J Urol 2002; 167: 2377–239

Kourambas J, Byrne RR, Preminger GM. Does a ureteral access sheath facilitate ureteroscopy? J Urol 2001; 165: 789–793

5. Percutaneous Access (PCNL)

PERCUTANEOUS RENAL ACCESS

A good percutaneous access pivots around careful pre-procedural planning of the access route. This ensures a safe puncture and also one that will allow easy intrarenal navigation to all the stone-bearing calyces. A thorough knowledge of the normal and variant upper tract anatomy is essential, and this is discussed first followed by the planning and technical aspects of renal access.

RENAL ANATOMY

Embryological development of the renal collecting system

This commences in the 5th week of gestation and continues up till the 34th week. First the metanephric duct grows upwards from the metanephric ridge, ascending from the fetal pelvis to the upper retroperitoneum and dividing to become the ureter, renal pelvis, calyces and collecting ducts. Ascend is accompanied by rotation of the kidney, and this sequence is illustrated in Figure 5.1. Development, ascend and/or rotation of the urinary tract may go awry at any stage and numerous variations of the normal urinary tract anatomy are feasible. The career endourologist should be able to recognise and be prepared for such variant collecting systems.

> DO! Be aware that anomalies of renal anatomy, ascend and orientation are common. Recognise them and modify your technique accordingly

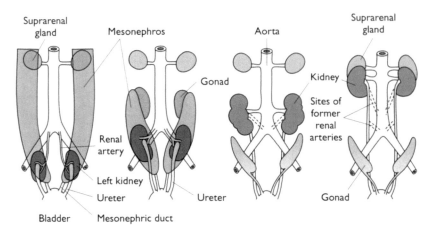

Figure 5.1 Normal ascend and rotation of the kidney. The kidneys develop in the fetal pelvis after the 5th week and ascend into their retroperitoneal position. The kidney also rotates antero-medially. Variations of ureteric and collecting ducts, ascend and arteries are common.

Position

The kidneys lie within the perinephric space, surrounded by the anterior and posterior lamina of the renal fascia (also called Gerota's fascia), at the level of T12 to L2/3 vertebral bodies. The upper pole of the kidneys lies more medial than the lower, at an axis tilt of about 15°. The upper pole is also more posterior facing than the lower. In the short axis the renal pelvis points antero-medially, as illustrated in Figure 5.1 and also Figure 4.10. This is the classical orientation (sometimes called the Brödel kidney), but variations are common. Examples of variations are: with age or inspiration the kidney 'falls' more inferiorly, the so-called ptotic kidney, and the upper pole flops more posteriorly, or in thin patients the antero-medial rotation of the renal pelvis is less pronounced, and so on. The common variations are listed in Box 5.1.

> **DO!** Remember that abnormalities of renal ascend, rotation and vascular maldevelopment often co-exist. For example, the horseshoe kidney is not only malascended and under-rotated, but will also have multiple and aberrant arterial vessels

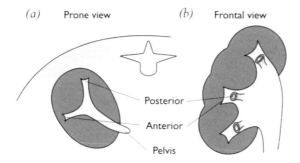

(a) Prone view   *(b)* Frontal view

Posterior

Anterior

Pelvis

Figure 5.2 Orientation of calyces in a 'normal' kidney. (a) Note that the pelvis faces antero-medially, and that calyces orientate anteriorly, posteriorly or in-between. (b) On a frontal view (like an IVU or fluoroscopic screen, image on the right) the posterior calyces are seen foreshortened and more medially placed.

Box 5.1 Variations in renal and ureteric anatomy

(1) Abnormalities of rotation
  - Over-rotated kidney – the pelvis points laterally
  - Under-rotated kidney – the short axis, and all the calyces, point posteriorly

(2) Abnormalities of ascend
  - Pelvic kidney – the long axis usually lies horizontally
  - Thoracic kidney – very rare

(3) Abnormalities of fusion
  - Horseshoe kidney – the kidney is malascended and under-rotated with a fixed bridge or isthmus
  - Crossed fused ectopia

(4) Ureteral anomalies
  - Bifid pelvis
  - Partial duplex
  - Complete duplex
  - Retro-caval or retro-iliac ureter

The relations of the kidney

Regarding percutaneous access of the kidney, the important relations are those adjacent structures that may be injured during track creation, e.g. the liver, spleen, diaphragm, pleura/lung and the colon, particularly with lateral punctures. Figure 5.3 illustrates the critical anatomical structures that lie close to the kidney and should be avoided. Variant anatomy should also be remembered, for example the splenic flexure of the descending colon may be abnormally high and posterior, and may be pierced during left renal puncture.

> TIP! If there is concern about injury to adjacent structures during track creation, get a CT scan to define the retroperitoneal anatomy. But this should be acquired in the prone position

The intrarenal or pelvi-calyceal anatomy of the kidney

The adult kidney has about eight or nine calyces and typically the upper and lower pole calyces undergo more fusion and these larger calyces are termed compound calyces, unlike the smaller interpolar calyces, called simple calyces (see Box 5.2). For the purposes of percutaneous access the larger, compound calyces are easier to access and navigate. However, it should be

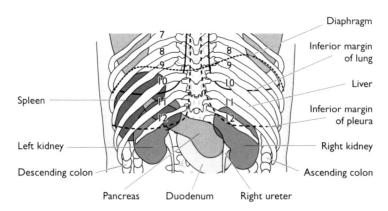

Figure 5.3 Posterior view showing the relationships of the kidney to surrounding structures that may be injured during PCNL. Note that the upper pole is covered by ribs. The pleura veers away from the ribs laterally and needle entry above the latter half of the 12th rib is safer (particularly during deep expiration). However, the spleen, liver and colon may be injured with a too lateral puncture.

Box 5.2 Simple or compound calyces?

- Simple calyx – one calyx draining into a single small infundibulum
- Compound calyx – many calyces fuse before draining into a single large infundibulum

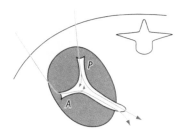

Figure 5.4 Posterior view showing how posterior calyces (P) allow easier inspection of the pelvis and other calyces (it's all downhill), unlike anterior calyx (A) entry.

remembered that the calyces will also vary in their orientation. Some calyces will face anteriorly, others will point posteriorly and yet others will be in-between. This variation in calyceal orientation is one of the most important factors to consider when planning renal access.

Naturally, the posterior calyx is ideal as it is closer to the skin surface in the prone position. Posterior calyces are always better for navigation purposes, for example the route from a posterior to an adjacent anterior calyx or the renal pelvis is more or less in a straight line forward. These points are illustrated in Figure 5.4.

OTHER ANATOMICAL FACTORS OF IMPORTANCE DURING PCNL ACCESS

Relationship to ribs and the pleura

Part of either kidney will lie above the 12th rib and even the 11th rib. This is more likely with the left kidney. Thus for access to the upper pole calyces intercostal puncture may be necessary. The particular hazard presented by supra 11th/12th rib puncture is intercostal artery or pleural injury.

The intercostal artery runs in a groove underneath the rib and may be damaged if needle entry is close to the lower surface, especially if angled cephalad. Regarding the pleura, it should be remembered that the posterior reflection of the parietal pleura lies horizontally, and is reflected off the 12th and the 11th ribs in its lateral portion. Thus a puncture through the latter half of the 12th or

11th intercostal space is safer as it avoids puncture of the parietal pleura. These key aspects of rib and pleural anatomy are illustrated in Figure 5.3.

TIP! Either maximal expiration or inspiration can help during percutaneous access

- Maximal expiration is safer for punctures above the ribs as the lungs are deflated superiorly
- However, maximal inspiration can push the kidney sufficiently downwards such that the upper pole comes to lie below the 12th rib

---

Renal vascular anatomy

The renal artery arises at T12–L1 level and divides into anterior and posterior portions. The anterior is the dominant division, and supplies the lower pole and anterior surface. It divides into three or four segmental branches that further divide into lobar and arcuate arteries. The posterior division usually continues as a single segmental branch to the upper pole and it should be remembered that this branch is the only major renal arterial division that lies posterior to the collecting system. Typically, it lies posteriorly at the level of the upper pelvis, but occasionally it is higher than this and runs behind the upper pole infundibulum, where it may be injured if upper pole entry is made through the infundibulum rather than the calyx. Figure 5.5 demonstrates the branches of the renal artery and their relationship to the calyces and how this influences the choice of renal access.

Normally there is a single renal artery and vein, but 20–25% of kidneys have more than one renal artery and variant renal veins are seen in 3–17%. These do not directly influence choice of access, but may explain the occasional vascular injury that occurs despite adherence to safe anatomical principles.

How renal anatomy influences percutaneous entry

From the above discussion it can be appreciated that there are numerous factors to consider when planning safe, effective percutaneous renal access for nephrolithotomy. The important considerations are summarised in Box 5.3.

A lower pole, postero-lateral puncture of the centre of the calyx is theoretically the safest. The upper pole is more posterior and allows for easier navigation but has to be approached with due care.

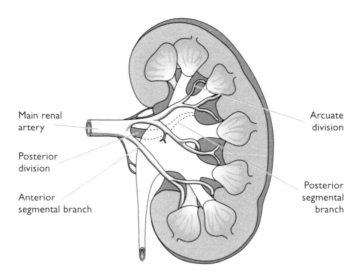

Main renal
artery

Posterior
division

Anterior
segmental branch

Arcuate
division

Posterior
segmental
branch

Figure 5.5 Anterior view of the renal arterial supply. Note the large posterior division artery and that it is safest to puncture the centre of a calyx approached laterally.

RENAL ACCESS

Over the years many different methods of renal access and sheath placement have been described. The commonest or 'usual' method is described below followed by some discussion of alternative methods. The equipment necessary is listed in Box 5.4 and a percutaneous access set is shown in Figure 5.6.

General principles

Choosing the calyx for renal access

The calyx chosen for puncture should be selected after careful appreciation of the collecting system anatomy and the position of stone/s within it. The chosen calyx should allow easy and maximal visualisation of the pelvis/upper ureter and as many of the calyces as possible. With careful choice, at the end of the PCNL all or the maximum amount of the stone should have been retrieved without losing fragments down the ureter. In most cases a single access will achieve this, but in a minority (e.g. complete staghorn) more than one track may be necessary. Again the need for more than one track should be predictable if the preliminary imaging is well studied, in which case all the

---

Box 5.3 Anatomical considerations that influence PCNL access in a 'normal' kidney

---

(1) The lie of the kidney:
- The upper pole is more posterior
- The short axis lies postero-laterally

(2) The calyces
- Lie either anterior or posterior
- Upper or lower calyces are often compound or fused and so bigger

(3) Vascular
- There is a theoretically 'avascular' line along the lateral margin of the kidney
- The lobar branches course in a curvilinear fashion around the calyx and papilla
- The posterior segmental division may lie behind the upper pole infundibulum

(4) Adjacent structures
- Pleura – lies above the 12th and 11th laterally
- Intercostal artery – underneath the rib
- Liver, spleen and (left) colon may overlie the upper pole

---

tracks can be made at the beginning of the procedure and time saved. There are some general rules that can help regarding the choice of calyx to puncture, and these are pictorially summarised in Figure 5.7.

Targeting the calyx for entry

The safest point for calyceal puncture is the centre of the calyx, approached through the relatively avascular plane (Brödel's line) between the branches of the anterior and posterior divisions of the renal artery. Puncturing the centre of the calyx avoids injury to the arcuate divisions that course around the infundibulum. This is the ideal and is illustrated in Figure 5.8; however in some cases infundibular entry is necessary, for example if the stone is tightly lodged in the calyx.

Box 5.4 Equipment necessary for initial renal access

Entry needle	Guidewires	Catheters
The choice is wide (1) 22 Access systems (e.g. Accustick, Boston Scientific) (2) 4F/5F Sheathed, diamond tip needle (e.g. Kellett, Longdwell or Leigen needle) (3) 18G Nephrostomy needle (diamond tip preferred) (We prefer a sheathed needle)	Choice is again wide (1) 0.018 inch platinum tipped, nitinol wire (2) 0.035 inch J tip stainless steel wire (3) 0.035 inch J tip hydrophilic wire (e.g. Terumo wire) (4) 0.035 inch Bentson wire (5) 0.035 inch Amplatz type super-stiff wire (We prefer a 0.035 inch hydrophilic wire for initial entry, and a 0.035 inch Amplatz super-stiff wire for dilatation)	5–6F shaped tipped catheter (e.g. Cobra, Kumpe, Biliary manipulation, etc.)

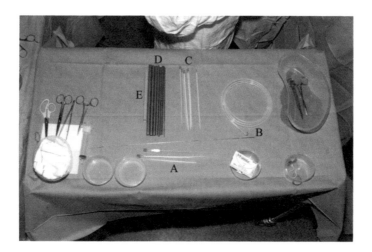

Figure 5.6 An operative tray prepared for percutaneous access for PCNL.
A = Access needles; B = J tipped wire; C = plastic dilators (the full set is not shown here); D = telescopic metal dilators; E = working sheath.

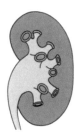

Principles of PCNL access
Aims
1 Aim for complete stone clearance.
2 If complete clearance is not possible:
   • Clear renal pelvis to improve renal drainage.
   • Clear lower pole calyces as these may not respond to ESWL.
   • Residual stones in the upper/interpolar calyces can later be treated with ESWL.
Renal access
1 Posterior calyces allow access to anterior calyces.
2 Anterior calyceal entry poorer for intra-renal navigation.
3 Upper pole entry allows deep access of the PUJ/upper ureter.
   • May puncture posterior division artery
   • May puncture pleura.
4 Some inter-polar calyces may be difficult with either lower or upper entry.

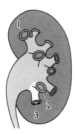

Lower pole branched calculus
Stones in anterior and posterior parallel calyces. Complete clearance as ESWL may not work.
1 Route 1 preferred as both parallel calyces well seen.
2 Route 2 (posterior calyx) better than 3 (anterior calyx) as navigation easier.

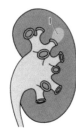

Stone in calyceal diverticulum with tight neck
Complete clearance is ideal. To decrease chances of recurrence, the neck should be dilated (thereby improving drainage) or the diverticulum should be obliterated. Direct puncture onto stone. Hydrophylic wire and good distension (with air/CO_2) help in searching for neck.
Intra-renal approach is possible – needle within diverticulum and injection of methylene blue help retrograde identification of neck.

Stone in renal pelvis
Stone removed with minimal fragmentation. Ureteric fragments may be difficult to chase. Access planned according to PUJ anatomy.

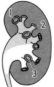

Stone in pelvis and lower calyces
Complete clearance is important (see under Principles–Aims).

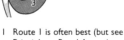

Complete staghorn
Stone clearance may be impossible with a single puncture.

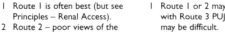

1 Routes 1 and 2 are preferred with straight navigation to PUJ.
2 Route 3 may be difficult if the infundibulo-pelvic angle is acute and distal stone may be beyond reach.

1 Route 1 is often best (but see Principles – Renal Access).
2 Route 2 – poor views of the interpolar calyx.
3 Route 3 – poor views of upper ureter.

1 Route 1 or 2 may be preferred – with Route 3 PUJ/ureteric clearance may be difficult.
2 With either routes some interpolar calyces may be difficult.

Figure 5.7 Line drawings illustrating the principles of renal access for PCNL (top row) and how these principles are applicable to the various stone configurations and dispositions commonly encountered. Figure reproduced from Sandhu C, Anson KM, Patel U. Urinary tract stones-part II: current status of treatment. Clin radiol 2003; 58:422–33, with permission.

Targeting and guiding the needle through this safe path to the calyx can be carried out under ultrasound or fluoroscopic guidance (rarely CT guidance may be necessary, e.g. for pelvic kidneys, see below). Fluoroscopy is the most commonly used and is described first.

PLANE OF ARTERIAL DIVISION

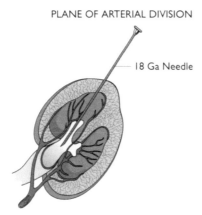

18 Ga Needle

Figure 5.8 It is safest to puncture the centre of a calyx approached laterally, as it minimises the risk of injury to large arterial divisions.

Fluoroscopically guided PCNL renal access

Selecting the calyx

First the collecting system is opacified using iodinated radiographic contrast medium. This is most commonly introduced by retrograde injection through a ureteric catheter placed cystoscopically. Further methods are the use of intravenous contrast media or ultrasound guidance.

DO! In the absence of a retrograde catheter, a 22G fine needle can be directed onto the stone under fluoroscopy and used to inject contrast

---

Contrast is injected until the target calyx is seen to opacify. Once seen, the orientation of the calyx can be verified. One fairly reliable rule is that the more medial calyces seen in a frontal projection are the posterior facing calyces (see Box 5.5). If the orientation is still in doubt, then rotation of the fluoroscopic arm can help. The calyces should be observed during continuous fluoroscopy as the arm is moved along an arc from $+30°$ to $-30°$. The

---

Box 5.5 Are the calyces posterior or anterior?

A good mnemonic to remember is LAMP:

* **L**ateral calyces are **A**nterior
* **M**edial calyces are **P**osterior

TIP! **How to identify a posterior calyx**

- The more medial calyces on an IVU or frontal fluoroscopic image are usually posterior (this rule is said to apply in 75% of kidneys)
- On rotating the C-arm the posterior calyces show a greater range of movement
- Air/CO_2 preferentially fills the posterior calyces (if the patient is in the prone position). **But it should be used with care:**
  - Inject gas slowly (<20 ml in total)
  - Make sure there is no possibility of intravasation
  - Inject under continuous fluoroscopy, so that lucent gas-filled calyces are not confused with bowel gas

calyces which show the most movement will be the most posterior (they move most because they are farther away from the X-ray source, which is usually under the table).

However, one of the limitations of using iodinated contrast for opacification is its relative density. In the prone position the contrast medium preferentially gravitates into the anterior calyces. Consequently the posterior calyces are only poorly seen. Double contrast pyelography (the use of air or CO_2 with iodinated contrast medium) substantially improves the appreciation of posterior calyces, but requires careful use. The principles are illustrated in Figure 5.9.

Targeting and puncturing the selected calyx

Once selected, the chosen calyx should be positioned for puncture. For accurate fluoroscopic guidance it should be placed scrupulously in the iso-centre of the radiographic monitor. This is termed iso-centricity (working in the centre of the beam). It is a central concept during fluoroscopic guidance and ensures that the errors due to beam divergence are minimised. Figures 5.10–5.11 explain how poor positioning can result in a substantial miscalculation of the needle path.

DO! Always maintain iso-centricity during needle puncture

Of course, if the fluoroscopic arm is in a strict antero-posterior position the needle will enter the calyx at a relatively unfavourable angle as the direc-

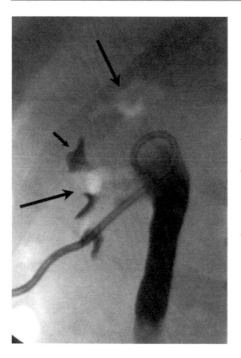

Figure 5.9 Double contrast pyelogram taken in the prone position. Introduced air has risen into posterior facing calyces seen as lucent (long arrows) compared to the anterior facing calyces that are seen filled with iodinated contrast (medium arrow). From this information the stone in the upper third of the ureter (seen as a filling defect in the ureter at the bottom of the picture) was removed by PCNL carried out via an upper pole puncture. As demonstrated double contrast pyelography helps in deciding which calyceal puncture will allow the easiest endoscopic navigation to the target stone.

tion of the infundibulum will be angled away and not straight ahead. For this reason a slightly angled needle entry is preferred. To achieve this the fluoroscopic arm should be angled slightly, depending on whether the upper, interpolar or lower pole calyx is being targeted. This principle of improving the direction of entry so that navigation is more favourable is explained in Figures 5.12–5.13.

> TIP! A slightly angled calyceal entry results in a PCNL track that favours intrarenal navigation

By angling the C-arm as described in Figures 5.12 and 5.14, the calyx will be seen in the iso-centre and the needle is positioned so that the calyx, the tip and the hub of the needle are all in the line – seen as a 'bull's eye' on fluoroscopy. The needle is advanced in small increments, all the while maintaining the bull's eye trajectory. Soon (after 7–10 cm length of the needle has been inserted) the needle tip will be seen to move in unison with the kidney and calyx during respiration. This means the needle has just penetrated the capsule and is 2–3 cm short of the calyx. Needle advancement can be continued until the calyx is reached, but as the depth of the calyx is not known

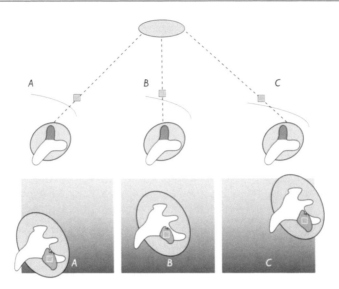

Figure 5.10 *A line illustration demonstrating the importance of isocentricity during renal puncture. The first row shows the abdomen in cross-section and the next row the corresponding view as seen on the monitor. In each case a marker (small orange squares) has been placed on the skin to overlie the target posterior calyx (coloured red) of the fluoroscopic image (as seen in the box). Although in all three images (A, B, C) it may seem that the calyx is directly vertical beneath the marker, only when the target is in the centre of the monitor and beam (that is iso-centric, image B) is this assumption correct. With the other two positions the marking is 'incorrect' because of beam divergence. Briefly, the target should* **always be in the centre of the screen**.

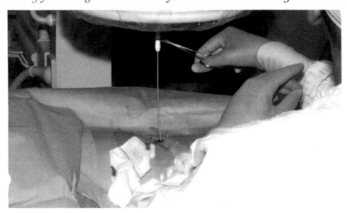

Figure 5.11 *An image demonstrating iso-centric needle positioning. Care should be taken to ensure that the needle and target are scrupulously placed in the centre of the image and hence the fluoroscopic beam. This ensures accurate targeting and is a key step in fluoroscopic guided intervention. (Note also how with the use of an arterial forceps to grip the needle shaft, the operator's hand can be maintained outside the radiation beam).*

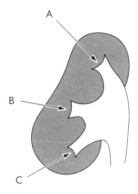

A – Upper pole pucture
- Approach at 10–20° medial and caudal direction

B – Interpolar puncture
- Approach at 10–20° medial

C – Lower pole puncture
- Approach at 10–20° medial and cephalad

Figure 5.12 Angling the direction of needle entry for more favourable calyceal entry and navigation. This diagram illustrates that with an upper pole entry the needle should be angled caudally, as this line of entry (track route) will favour caudally directed navigation towards the pelvis and lower pole calyces. Conversely, with lower pole entry the needle should be angled relatively cephalad, and with an interpolar puncture the needle should be directed relatively medially.

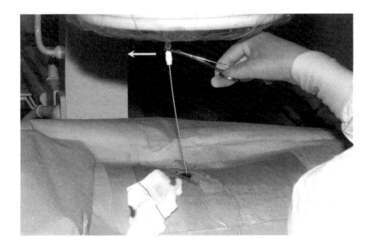

Figure 5.13 In this image the needle is being angled in a cranio-caudal direction (arrow) to improve the angle of entry into an upper pole calyx (refer to Figure 5.12).

this requires some guesswork. To decide more accurately the depth of needle entry necessary, the C-arm should be rotated directly away (about 20° angulation away is usually sufficient). By this means the depth of the calyx becomes apparent and the needle can be advanced to just within the calyx. Figure 5.14 illustrates the entire sequence for gaining fluoroscopically guided percutaneous renal access in a stepwise fashion.

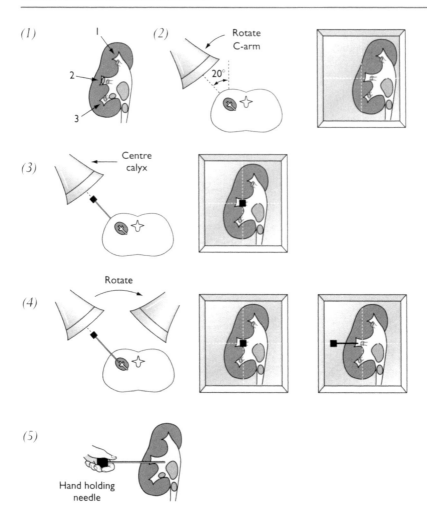

Figure 5.14 (1) The calyx is chosen according to stone location (calyx 2 for this illustration). (2) The C-arm is moved to 20° near-oblique position (with additional cranial or cephalad movement as necessary – see Figure 5.12) to allow an angled calyceal entry. (3) The C-arm is shifted so the target calyx is seen iso-centric and the needle hub as a 'bulls-eye', the needle slowly advanced (1 cm increments) using intermittent fluoroscopy, all the while maintaining iso-centricity and the bulls-eye view. (4) When the needle is seen to move with the kidney, the C-arm is moved to 20° far-obliquity. The needle image is seen to change from a bulls-eye to an angled view. The needle tip is just within/short of the calyx and requires final adjustment. (5) The side-to-side shutters are closed so that the hand on the needle hub is not in the radiation beam, and under continuous fluoroscopy the needle is advanced the final 1–2 cm into the calyx.

However, the calyx can be surprisingly tough and the needle may deviate off trajectory at the last moment of calyceal puncture. Just a few degrees' deviation can veer the needle sufficiently off target. If final confirmation is required that the needle is within the calyx and has not veered off, then the C-arm should be slowly rotated in an arc from $+30°$ to $-20°$ (see Box 5.6).

Box 5.6 Parallax

If the needle is within the calyx, on rotating the C-arm the needle tip and the calyx will move in unison and always be seen close together. If their positions diverge then the needle is not in the calyx. This basic fluoroscopic principle is called parallax and is illustrated in Figure 5.15

If needle position is satisfactory then urine should flow on removal of the central obturator. However, this may not happen if the calyx is filled with air/CO_2. Retrograde injection of contrast through the ureteric catheter may help. Avoid injecting contrast down the sheath to confirm position, as this may obscure the vision if contrast extravosates. Use saline instead and watch for diluting of existing contrast in the renal pelvis. If doubt continues, then a

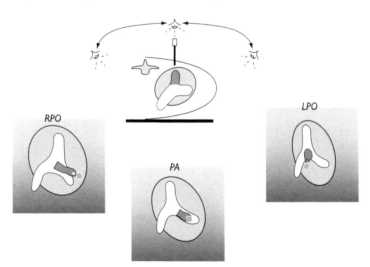

Figure 5.15 Line illustration demonstrating how the shifting relationships between structures on C-arm rotation can help to evaluate the spatial relationship of structures. In this example in all three images the relationship between the needle tip and target posterior calyx (coloured red) stays constant because these two points are iso-centric in 3D space. RPO = Right posterior oblique; PA = Posterior-anterior; LPO = Left posterior oblique.

hydrophilic wire is advanced down the sheath with a gentle probing motion. If the sheath is in the calyx the wire can be manipulated into the renal pelvis.

DON'T! Contrast is best not injected down the needle sheath as this will obscure the view in the event of extravasation

---

Is the needle in the calyx?

DO! Inject saline and watch for dilution
DO! If doubt continues use a hydrophilic wire with a gentle probing motion

---

Ultrasound guided PCNL

If ultrasound is used to guide the needle, the method is very similar. However, some time should be taken to evaluate the calyceal anatomy and choose the best calyx for entry, using the principles illustrated in Figure 5.7. This is more difficult than with fluoroscopy and should be done with reference to a pre-operative IVU to evaluate the intrarenal anatomy. Three-dimensional ultrasound is still too crude for this purpose.

TIP! Use a pre-operative IVU (or CT) to map the intrarenal anatomy and choose the best calyx to puncture under US guidance

---

Once the calyx is selected, a ureteric catheter is used to distend the collecting system with saline and the needle is directed under real-time guidance into the centre of the calyx, along the avascular Brödel's line. For guidance either a dedicated needle guide is used or a freehand technique; the latter requires some experience as the two hands of the operator (one holding the guide and the other directing the needle) have to be kept strictly aligned in one plane. Once the needle is felt to be within the calyx, wire advancement and the remainder of the procedure are carried out under fluoroscopic guidance.

Track dilatation

Securing the wire to support dilatation

The kidney is a tough, mobile organ that resists dilatation. A stiff, straight wire path makes dilatation much easier. Time spent in securing a stiff wire is always rewarded. The hydrophilic wire should be exchanged for an Amplatz super-stiff wire. This rigid wire will orientate the calyx, infundibulum, the renal pelvis and the ureter into a straight path without acute angles. This avoids kinking of the wire during dilatation. Counsel of perfection is that at this stage a second safety wire should be inserted through a dual lumen catheter/sheath.

> **DO!** A stiff wire down the ureter and curled in the bladder is the most secure for dilatation

> **DO!** Have a safety wire in place

Next, a 1 cm long incision is made around the stiff wire and the track dilated using telescopic metal dilators (Figure 5.16), sequential Teflon® (Amplatz) dilators or a balloon dilator (see Chapter 3 for technical details of this equipment and their use). The methods and merits of each method are summarised in Table 5.1.

Once the track has been dilated the working sheath (this can be 24–34F) is advanced using a rotating method (Figure 5.17).

> **DO!** Dilate using a rotatory motion with slow advancement

> **DO!** If the calyx is stone bearing, dilate only up to the calyx and not beyond, otherwise the stone will fragment and some pieces may go down the ureter

> **DON'T!** If the infundibulum is narrow do not advance the dilators/sheath across the infundibulum as this will tear the urothelium

Table 5.1 Three methods of dilatation are in common use, and their merits and disadvantages are summarised here

	Advantages	Disadvantages
Metal	• Cheap and re-usable • Zero-tip dilatation • Can cope with tough tissues • Can be used to improve orientation of the kidney	• Slower • Linear (shear) force • Can puncture pelvis
Amplatz	• Smooth profile • Disposable	• Cost • Not zero-tip • Linear and radial force (linear force is a shearing force)
Balloon	• Quick • Radial dilatation	• Requires more secure access, as not zero-tip, so not suitable for calyceal diverticulum or if wire coiled in calyx • Cost

---

DON'T! Try and push a dilator over a kinked guidewire as this will tear the collecting system

---

DON'T! Overadvance the working sheath over the dilator/balloon as this may puncture the renal pelvis

---

Technical difficulties during needle access and dilatation

Most percutaneous renal access procedures are straightforward if the principles outlined above regarding careful planning of trajectory and calyceal entry are followed. However, in a minority problems may be encountered, most of which are solvable if recognised. Box 5.7 lists the various difficulties

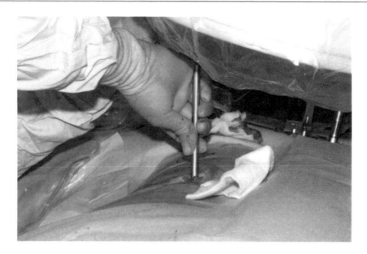

Figure 5.16 *Metal dilators are being used to dilate a track for PCNL. Note the position of the hands of the operator. This allows the operator to dilate with mostly rotatory action and slow forward advancement. This way the likelihood of trauma, and particularly pelvic perforation, is decreased. Note also that the fluoroscopic beam has been angled away so that the dilatation can be carried out under continuous fluoroscopy without radiating the operator's hands (this is the same principle as explained in Figure 5.14, under step 5).*

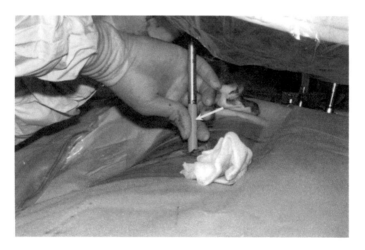

Figure 5.17 *A track has been dilated and a 30F working sheath (arrow) is being advanced over a 30F metal dilator. The sheath is poorly radio-opaque and careful technique is required to advance it just into the target and not leave it short.*

Box 5.7 Trouble shooting difficulties during renal access

(1) Mobile kidney – place a bolster underneath the patient to fix the kidney. Use a stiff wire. Use a balloon dilator

(2) Kink in wire – best is to exchange for a new wire. If this isn't possible, advance the kink down the ureter (but careful you don't damage the pelvis/ureter) or pull the kink back until it is external to the patient (but watch you don't lose access)

(3) Parallel lie – use a Y-puncture or make a new entry

(4) Staghorn/tight system – use the ureteric catheter to distend and a hydrophilic wire. If wire will not advance past the stone, coil tip in the calyx if possible and dilate with care

(5) Stone tightly in calyx and wire won't pass – as above, or puncture another calyx and approach the stone internally

(6) Pelvic/infundibular tear – there is a danger of absorption or retroperitoneal collection of irrigant. Procedure can continue with care but proper post-operative drainage should be ensured

(7) Brisk bleeding – place a balloon and tamponade the track. If bleeding continues consider open surgical repair or embolisation

---

commonly encountered during these procedures, how they may be avoided and corrected.

Difficult renal access

Sometimes a modified access may be more useful and anomalies of renal development or ascent also require a customised approach, but any kidney can be successfully accessed if approached with a proper understanding of the anatomy. The following list explains the modifications required for establishment of percutaneous access in these cases, and should be read in conjunction with Chapter 9, which further expands on difficult percutaneous nephrolithotomy.

(1) **Upper pole punctures:** The advantages of upper pole entry are that as it is more posterior entry is easier, navigation down to the PUJ simple and even the upper half of the ureter is accessible as the navigation route is more or less 'downhill'. The disadvantages are that an intercostal puncture is often necessary with the risk of pleural or intercostal artery damage and there is the possibility of puncturing the posterior division of the renal artery, which

lies behind the upper pole infundibulum. Further disadvantages are post-operative pain, etc., from pleural and intercostal muscle irritation. With careful technique these can all be minimised. The calyx should be carefully entered in the centre and the puncture path should follow the outer half of the intercostal space to minimise pleural injury. Maximal expiration reduces the chance of lung injury, but this may move the kidney even higher. Sometimes, maximal inspiration is better as this may push the upper pole calyx below the 12th rib, allowing a subcostal entry.

> **DO!** The puncture path should follow the outer half of the intercostal space to minimise pleural injury

> **DO!** Get a post-operative CXR to exclude lung/pleural injury

> **DO!** Consider an intercostal nerve block or patient controlled post-operative analgesia if an intercostal entry route is used

(2) **Horseshoe kidney:** the anatomical hazards with a horseshoe kidney are that it is an under-rotated and malascended kidney, with numerous accessory arteries. Furthermore, fusion of the two kidneys means that it is relatively immobile, which hinders intrarenal navigation. Pre-operative 3D CT is of particular help here for access planning. As a general rule the upper pole, medial calyces are preferred, and the use of double-contrast pyelography is very useful in identifying the most posterior calyces.

> **DO!** Long sheaths may be necessary as the horseshoe is usually more deeply located

(3) **Malrotated kidneys:** a kidney may be over- or under-rotated with the posterior calyces facing medially or laterally. There may also be anomalous vessels present. In this situation a CT scan with 3D volume reconstruction is very helpful. This helps to clarify the calyceal anatomy and its relation with the vessels.

(4) **Calyceal diverticulum:** most are stone packed and in the upper pole. The particular difficulty is that, although the needle can be readily targeted

onto the stone, the wire will either not enter the diverticulum, because of lack of space, or if it does it cannot be manipulated across the tight calyceal neck and down the ureter. Firm retrograde injection can help to distend both the neck and the diverticulum, but usually it is only with patience and a well lubricated hydrophilic wire that the tip can be manipulated across the neck. Once this is accomplished dilatation is straightforward. If the wire will not pass through the neck then it should be coiled firmly within the diverticulum and dilatation carried out with the utmost care and slowly.

DO! Use metal dilators, especially if wire access is poor, because they are zero-tip systems that allow accurate dilatation up to the diverticulum without disrupting the neck

---

(5) **Bifid or duplex systems:** the importance here is to recognise these anomalies and that navigation will be restricted. Such systems are also overall 'small' and prone to calyceal tearing during dilatation.

DO! Entry should be directly onto the stone-bearing calyx

---

(6) **Pelvic or thoracic kidneys:** pre-operative CT is a must here and percutaneous entry may require CT guidance or laparoscopic assistance to move away interposed bowel loops or lungs.

SUGGESTED FURTHER READING

Castaneda-Zuniga WR, Brady TM, Thomas R, et al. Percutaneous uroradiologic techniques. In Castaneda-Zuniga WR, Tadavarthy SM, Qian Z, Ferral H, Mayanr M, eds. Interventional Radiology. Baltimore: Williams and Wilkins, 1997: 1049–270

Marcovich R, Smith AD. Percutaneous renal access: tips and tricks. BJU Int 2005; 95: 78–84

Sampaio FJB. Renal collecting system anatomy: its possible role in the effectiveness of renal stone treatment. Curr Op Urol 2001; 11: 359–66

Sandhu C, Anson K, Patel U. Urinary tract stones – part 2: current status of treatment. Clin Rad 2003; 58: 422–33

Wong MC. An update on percutaneous nephrolithotomy in the management of urinary calculi. Curr Op Urol 2001; 11: 367–72

Part II
Clinical Aspects

6. UNEXPLAINED UPPER TRACT HAEMATURIA

Macroscopic haematuria is a common clinical problem; in those with an underlying cause, urine culture and cytology, routine upper tract imaging and cystoscopy are diagnostic. In the rest the haematuria remains unexplained and does not recur. However, there are a few patients with unilateral supravesical bleeding in whom these initial investigations are normal and the bleeding is recurrent. While common conditions, including renal cell carcinoma, transitional cell carcinoma (TCC) of the renal pelvis or ureter (Figure

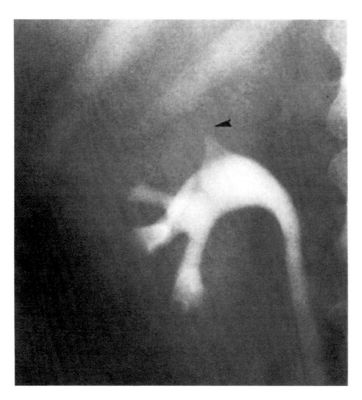

Figure 6.1 *IVU demonstrating cut-off of the upper pole infundibulum (arrowhead) that may be secondary to inflammation, infection or neoplasia. Retrograde ureterography and ureterorenoscopy will help establish diagnosis.*

6.1) and renal or ureteric calculus may still be the cause of bleeding, less common conditions must be considered. Table 6.1 lists causes of supravesical haematuria.

Table 6.1 Causes of unilateral supravesical haematuria

Congenital	Acquired
Arteriovenous malformations	Upper tract transitional cell carcinoma
Bleeding diathesis	Renal cell carcinoma
Congenital haemoglobinopathy	Calculi
Klippel–Trenaunay syndrome	Endometriosis
Renal haemangioma	Renal arteriopelvic fistula
Renal vein hypertension	Renal arteriovenous fistula
(secondary to venous and arterial anomalies, renal ptosis and aberrant peripheral nerve)	(can be spontaneous, traumatic, iatrogenic)
	Renal papillary necrosis
	Renal tuberculosis
	Renal vein hypertension
	(secondary to previous retroperitoneal surgery, unilateral idiopathic retroperitoneal fibrosis, primary haematuria of glomerular origin)
	Lesions of papilla – renal papilla varices, rupture of dilated veins in papillae
	Haemorrhagic papillitis
	Renal forniceal haemorrhage

BENIGN LATERALISING HAEMATURIA

Frank haematuria that is unilateral and supravesical in origin which cannot be diagnosed by routine radiological, cytological or haematological investigations is known as benign lateralising haematuria (BLH) (See Box 6.1). Other terms used to describe this condition include benign essential haematuria, lateralising essential haematuria and chronic unilateral haematuria.

BLH is a diagnostic and therapeutic challenge. As first- and second-line investigations fail to identify a suitable cause for the bleeding, ureterorenoscopy (URS) assumes a pivotal role in diagnosis and therapy. URS usually identifies the bleeding to be emanating from a vascular lesion in the kidney, and through a combination of direct vision and biopsy, malignant lesions are ruled out. This is in contrast to the days prior to ureteroscopy, when failure to identify a cause in the presence of chronic haematuria would eventually lead to partial or total nephrectomy.

Box 6.1 Clinical features of BLH

- No predisposition to any particular age, sex or side
- Patients may suffer with renal colic due to clot formation
- Haematuria can be severe enough to cause anaemia
- Patients may need blood transfusion

DON'T! Of primary concern to both the urologist and patient is that a cancer is not missed

Aetiology

BLH is a result of vascular lesions due to extrarenal or intrarenal vascular abnormalities. Most lesions can be diagnosed from their typical appearance (see Figures 6.2–6.3) Boxes 6.2, 6.3–6.4 describe the common vascular abnormalities seen at URS.

Box 6.2 Haemangioma

- May be congenital or acquired
- Most common vascular lesion causing BLH
- Usually large (range microscopic up to 10 cm in size; average 1–2 cm)
- May show up on angiography
- On flexi URS typically appears as a small red or bluish spot found at the tip or base of a papilla
- Mulberry-like in appearance
- Can be diffusely demarcated from surroundings

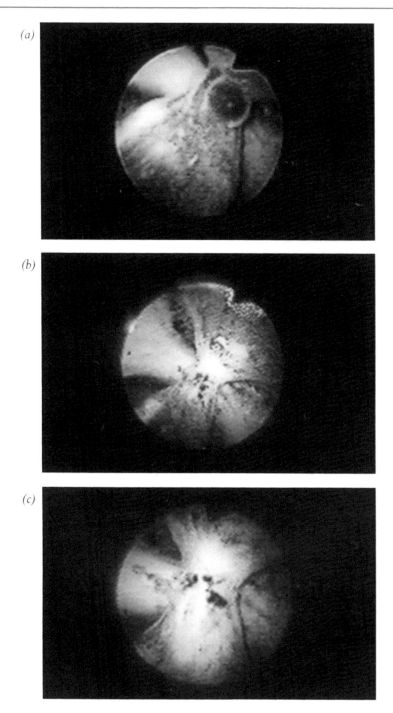

Figure 6.2 (a)Vascular abnormality on isthmus of a compound papilla seen at flexi URS; probable haemangioma. (b) and (c) Following Nd:YAG laser coagulation.

Box 6.3 Small lesions of renal papilla or fornix

- Disturbances of the vasculature of papillary and forniceal venous plexuses
- Include varices of the renal papilla, haemorrhagic papillitis, pyelo-venous fistula and renal forniceal haemorrhages
- Renal vein sinus-like tributaries in mucosa of fornix
- Rupture of dilated veins in renal papillae
- Direct communication (fistulae) between venous sinuses and calyces in the region of the calyceal fornix
- Venous–calyceal fistulae can be seen on IVU or retrograde imaging as pyelovenous backflow on retrograde

Box 6.4 Renal venous hypertension (RVH)

- Disturbances in renal haemodynamics in the calyceal fornices
- Leads to formation of venous–calyceal fistulae and bleeding
- Most commonly reported causes are venous anomalies like nut-cracker syndrome and left renal vein anomalies including persisting left inferior vena cava, retroaortic left renal vein and circumaortic left renal vein

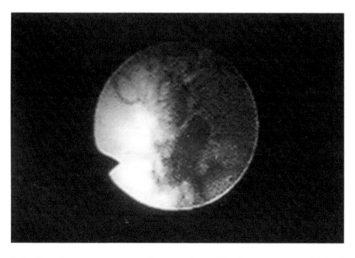

Figure 6.3 Vascular congestion at fornix of papilla. Patient stopped bleeding following this ureterorenoscopy.

INVESTIGATIONS

Routine first-line investigations for haematuria include voided urine for culture and cytology, flexible cystoscopy and imaging of the upper tracts with ultrasound and IVU. The IVU may reveal a filling defect (Figure 6.1). If the upper tract imaging is normal and cystoscopy reveals supravesical bleeding then Doppler studies may help elucidate the presence of a vascular malformation. If these investigations prove negative, then further urine and haematological tests are required (Box 6.5). In the event that this combination of investigations fails to yield a diagnosis, rigid cystoscopy followed by retrograde ureteropyelography, semi-rigid ureteroscopy and flexible ureterorenoscopy are undertaken.

Box 6.5 Second-line investigations for haematuria

Urine	*Serum*
Phase-contrast urine microscopy	Full blood count
• Dysmorphic red cells – indicates a glomerular source	Clotting studies
	Hb electrophoresis
• Normal red cells – anatomic lesion	Renal biochemistry
Urine analysis for proteinuria	Sickle cell if appropriate
• Non-glomerular source associated with an increase in HMW proteins	

ENDOSCOPIC DIAGNOSIS

Percutaneous and retrograde upper tract endoscopy has revolutionised the investigation and particularly the treatment of BLH. Initially, operative nephroscopy allowed bleeding to be localised to an individual calyx that could subsequently be removed by renal parenchymal-sparing surgery. With the advent of percutaneous nephroscopes, retrograde rigid and semirigid ureteroscopes and flexible ureterorenoscopes that incorporate a working-channel, endoscopic-treatment by fulguration and laser ablation became possible. Endoscopic access has also resulted in the discovery of new urothelial abnormalities that may be important in the pathogenesis of BLH.

Haemangiomas, TCC and calculi are causes of BLH in 24.8%, 5.1% and 3.7% of cases, respectively. Haemangiomas may appear either as small red or bluish spots at the tip or base of a papilla or as larger bulbous erythematous lesions on a papillary tip. TCCs, like submucosal haemangiomas, are readily identified endoscopically. However, diffuse inflammatory lesions can be confused with high-grade TCCs or TCCs of unusual appearance. Thus a biopsy should be taken from all lesions that are thought to be TCC or the appearances of which are inconclusive. Calculi are easily identified endoscopically.

> DO! **Take a biopsy!** Histology should always be obtained to confirm the diagnosis and avoid missing the rare case when a TCC can look like an inflammatory lesion

A pathological classification of these lesions has not yet been possible because only a few reported lesions have been biopsied before endoscopic treatment and the histological assessment of these has been disappointing. In the absence of histological evidence the responsibility of discrete endoscopic lesions for BLH has been inferred from the excellent outcomes obtained after ablative treatment. However, a direct causal relationship between these lesions and BLH cannot always be assumed because cases in which no abnormality was found at endoscopy have also been reported to have a good prognosis.

Discrete endoscopic lesions can be iatrogenic; for example a lesion at the base of an upper pole papilla may be caused by a guidewire advanced inadvertently, and hyperaemia can arise from contact between the endoscope and the urothelium or from overdistension (as in the bladder). Diffuse lesions may also represent the endoscopic appearances of the nutcracker phenomenon and other causes of RVH, although this condition does not always cause endoscopic abnormalities.

ACCURACY OF ENDOSCOPY IN BLH

In up to 16% of cases no endoscopic abnormality may be seen. Three possible explanations have been proposed to explain the absence of endoscopic lesions in patients with documented BLH. First, the endoscopic examination may have been incomplete. Endoscopic abnormalities have been reported in all three major groups of calyces and in the renal pelvis, making a complete examination of the entire pelvicalyceal system mandatory. The use of the new third-generation flexible fibreoptic ureterorenoscopes, incorporating a passively deflectable segment proximal to the actively deflectable distal segment, has resulted in an increase in the proportion of cases in which there was a complete examination, and a corresponding reduction in the proportion of cases with a negative endoscopy. Second, it was suggested that even with a complete examination, small lesions may be missed. Some investigators consider that the absence of active bleeding increases the chances of missing small lesions, as bleeding focuses the exploration and (because it is venous) can be controlled by varying the irrigation pressure so as not to obscure vision. Finally, it was suggested that venous–calyceal communications, too small to be visualised endoscopically, are responsible for BLH in cases where no abnormality can be found. The closure of these communications by the increased intrapelvic pressure or inflammation from the endoscopic procedure has been proposed to explain the therapeutic effect of endoscopy reported in some series in patients in whom no abnormality is discovered.

ENDOSCOPIC TREATMENT OF BLH

Endoscopic treatment is the mainstay of the management for BLH. Patients with discrete lesions are more amenable to treatment. Up to 50% of patients undergoing URS will have a discrete vascular lesion that can be treated (Table 6.2). Care must be taken during URS to avoid iatrogenic bleeding (see Box 6.2). Diathermy fulguration and laser ablation (Figure 6.2) are two effective treatments of discrete lesions.

Table 6.2 Discrete vs diffuse lesions on URS

	Discrete lesions	Diffuse lesions
Typical location	Calyces – papilla or fornix	Renal pelvis, infundibulae and calyces
Causes	Venous ruptures	Diffuse erythema
	Peripapillary varices	Inflammation
	Abnormal papillary tip	Hyperaemia
	Dilated collecting ducts	Diffuse petechiae

Box 6.6 Iatrogenic causes of bleeding during URS

- Guidewire – may cause bleeding at the papillae
- Irrigation – high pressures can cause bleeding at calyceal fornix
- Pelvis – overdistension of the renal pelvis may cause diffuse submucosal haemorrhages and non-specific erythema

Ureteroscopic technique

A methodical and skilled approach to upper tract endoscopy will lead to diagnostic confidence upon which the surgeon and patient can depend. The principles to follow are outlining the anatomy, systematic endoscopy of the entire urothelium on the involved side with minimal instrumentation and complete visualisation of all of the ureter and intrarenal collecting system without trauma. Box 6.7 outlines the key steps.

DO! The entire intrarenal collecting system should be inspected without prior instrumentation to avoid iatrogenic injury of urothelium

Box 6.7 Ureterorenoscopy for BLH: operative steps

(1) Retrograde ureteropyelography
(2) Draw a road map of the anatomy
(3) Semirigid URS examination without a guidewire up to the proximal ureter
(4) Guidewire inserted to the proximal ureter
(5) Flexi URS
(6) Low-pressure irrigation
(7) Inspect pelvis, upper, middle and lower poles (in that order)
(8) Ureteric stent if lots of bleeding and come back

Road map

The retrograde study provides the road map for the URS. Retrograde can be done using the ureteric catheter advanced into the first few centimetres of the distal ureter or can be performed via the semirigid ureteroscope. Once the ureter and calyces are displayed, an anatomical drawing must be made for the operator to refer to during the procedure (see Chapter 4, Figure 4.11). The calyces are numbered starting from the upper pole in a clockwise manner.

Semirigid URS

The 6.9F semirigid is slowly advanced to inspect up to the proximal ureter. It is important to have complete visualisation of the whole circumference of the lumen of the ureter. Once the semirigid scope has been passed to the furthest extent, a floppy-tip hydrophilic guidewire is inserted up to the tip of the endoscope, which is then removed over the wire.

Flexi URS

The smallest calibre flexible URS is inserted over the guidewire and advanced beyond to inspect the remaining proximal ureter and intrarenal collecting system (IRCS). The infundibulae and calyces are inspected in a systematic sequential pattern, starting with upper to middle to lower poles. Entry into all calyces must be confirmed on fluoroscopy and cross referenced with the drawn road map. Any positive findings should be indicated on the roadmap.

DO! Lower pole entry should be left to last. Entry may require contact with the mucosa at the mouth of the upper pole infundibulum, which can be traumatic

---

Irrigation

DO! Continuous irrigation should be maintained at minimum pressure as it will aid in examination of venous bleeding points
DO! Turn off the flow of irrigation to see bleeding from small haemangioma and venous ruptures
DO! Aspirate fluid through the flexi URS to reduce volume and pressure within the IRCS

Endoscopic treatment

The two main options are electrofulguration (Figure 6.4) and laser ablation. Diathermy fulguration is inexpensive and readily available. Coagulation can

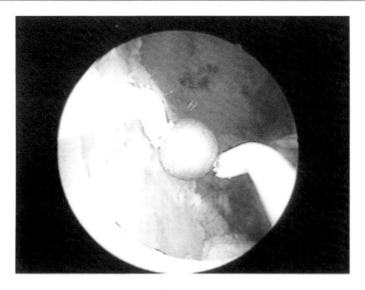

Figure 6.4 Percutaneous ablation of abnormal urothelium in the renal pelvis.

be performed via flexible URS using a 2 or 3F Greenwald blunt-tip electrode set at 40–50 W. Laser surgery is more expensive but is becoming more widely used. An advantage of laser ablation over electrosurgery is the ability to use isotonic saline instead of glycine for irrigation.

Both Nd:YAG and Ho:YAG lasers have been used in the upper tract for the treatment of vascular and inflammatory lesions in BLH. The Ho:YAG laser is delivered at 0.5–1.0 J/pulse and 5–10 pulse/s, whilst the Nd:YAG laser is used at powers of 15–30 W. Endoscopy in BLH is safe and there have been no reported perioperative deaths. Endoscopic treatment leads to success in at least 50% of patients (see Box 6.8).

Box 6.8 Results of endoscopic treatment of BLH

- Discrete lesions: up to 87% success (bleeding stops and does not return)
- Diffuse lesions: 58% success
- No lesion seen: overall supportive treatment results in 50% success

---

For treatment of vascular abnormalities the Nd:YAG is the preferred wavelength. It allows the area of concern to be coagulated to a depth of up to 8 mm in a non-contact mode. The Ho:YAG will vapourise the tissue requiring near contact which may result in further bleeding and an inability to fully treat the lesion. The complications of endoscopic treaatment are listed in Box 6.9.

Other treatment options

Epsilon aminocaproic acid can be given orally for short-term control of bleeding. However, treatment for at least 3 weeks is needed for any effect to be noticed. Retrograde lavage treatments used with success include lavage of the intrarenal collecting system with contrast medium, methylene blue, adrenaline and 10 ml silver nitrate (1%). In heavy bleeding, tamponade with a ureteric balloon catheter can be attempted. The last resort remains a nephrectomy (partial or total). An algorithm for the managment of BLH is provided in Figure 6.5.

Box 6.9 Complications of endoscopic management of BLH

- Urinary infection
- Clot colic
- Obstruction after premature removal of ureteric stents and catheters
- Extravasation of irrigant
- Ureteric stricture
- Failure to identify and treat abnormality

SUGGESTED FURTHER READING:

Lano MD, Wagoner RD, Leary FJ. Unilateral essential hematuria. Mayo Clin Proc 1979; 54: 8890

Nakada SY, Elashry OM, Picus D, Clayman RV. Long-term outcome of flexible ureterorenoscopy in the diagnosis and treatment of lateralizing essential hematuria. J Urol 1997; 157: 776–9

Rowbotham C, Anson KM. Benign lateralizing haematuria: the impact of upper tract endoscopy. BJU Int 2001; 88: 841–9

Tawfiek ER, Bagley DH. Ureteroscopic evaluation and treatment of chronic unilateral hematuria. J Urol 1998; 160: 700–2

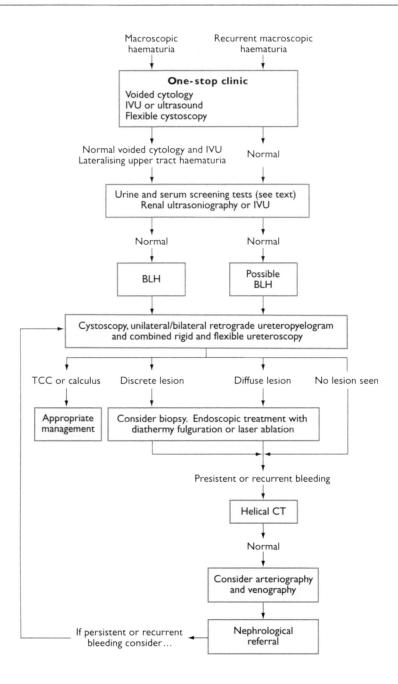

Figure 6.5 Algorithm for management of BLH. Reproduced from Rowbotham C, Anson KM. Benign lateralizing haematuria: the impact of upper tract endoscopy. BJU Int 2001; 88: 841–9, with permission.

7. URETERIC CALCULI

Urinary stones have afflicted humans for centuries and the first reported cases are bladder and renal calculi found in Egyptian mummies dated 4800 BC. The prevalence of the disease is between 2–3% and it is estimated that the likelihood of a Caucasian developing a stone by the age of 70 is approximately 1 in 8. Acute renal colic is a common, often recurrent condition with an annual incidence of 1–2 cases per 1000 and a lifetime risk of 10–20% for men and 3–5% for women. The last 30 years have seen a revolution in the surgical management of urinary stone disease, with the gradual disappearance of open stone surgery and the emergence of increasingly efficacious minimally invasive techniques.

The chances of passing a ureteric stone depend upon the size and location of the stone (Table 7.1). In the presence of normal anatomy, the majority of ureteric stones will pass spontaneously. Intervention is required when the stone fails to move, the patient has persistent pain, if the stone is larger than 5 mm, if renal function is at risk and if infection intervenes.

Table 7.1 Spontaneous passage of a ureteric stone according to site and size (AUA Guidelines 1997)

Site of stone	Size of stone	Spontaneous stone passage (%)
Proximal ureter	<5mm	29–98
	>5mm	10–53
Distal ureter	<5mm	71–98
	>5mm	25–53

Reproduced from Table 2, Sandhu et al. Urinary tract stones – Part II: current status of treatment. Clin Radiol 2003; 58: 422–33, with permission

Ureteric calculi (Figure 7.1) can be managed with a variety of modalities including ESWL, ureteroscopy, percutaneous techniques, laparoscopic or open surgery. Currently, the vast majority of stones are treated with ESWL and ureteroscopy. The choice between these depends upon the size and location of the stone, stone composition, renal function, whether associated obstruction or infection is present, patient factors (age, co-morbidity,

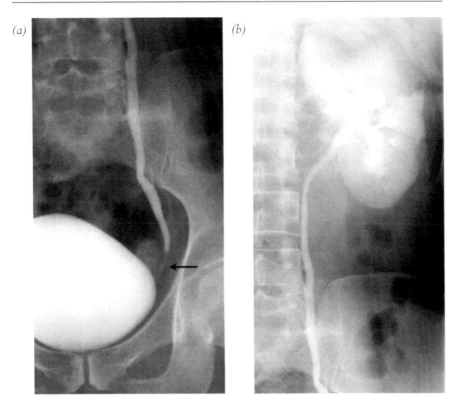

Figure 7.1 This montage of an IVU study shows a ureteric calculus in the lower third of the ureter resulting in acute ureteric obstruction. (a) Shows the calculus (arrowed) and (b) shows hydronephrosis and contrast extravasation due to rupture of a lower pole calyx. Although this presents a radiographically dramatic image, the presence of calyceal rupture is not, on its own, an indication for intervention.

body habitus), patient preference, experience/skill of the urologist and the availability of appropriate equipment.

ESWL has proven to be of great benefit for ureteric calculi and is now competing with ureterorenoscopy as the treatment of choice for the majority of ureteric calculi. The various pros and cons of each approach are listed in Table 7.2. If the cost and maintenance of ESWL are taken into account, ureteroscopic treatment of ureteric calculi (at all sites) has been shown to be more cost effective (Lotan et al., 2002). We will not be dealing with ESWL in any detail.

Table 7.2 ESWL or ureteroscopy?

ESWL	Ureteroscopy
• Non-invasive outpatient treatment requiring no general anaesthesia	• Superior overall stone-free rate especially for distal and mid-ureteric stones
• Equivalent to URS for calculi <5–10 mm	• Shorter treatment time
• Minimal morbidity	• Should be preferred choice for stones >1cm
• Few contraindications	• Longer hospitalisation and need for general anaesthesia
• Longer time to be stone free	• More minor complications
• Higher retreatment rates especially for mid-ureteric stones	

ENDOSCOPIC MANAGEMENT

Over the past 20 years there has been a remarkable progress in the development of small atraumatic ureteroscopes that has allowed easy access to all parts of the ureter. In conjunction with this there have been great advances in miniaturisation of intracorporeal lithotriptors and ancillary instruments. These advances have allowed urologists to treat calculi successfully throughout the ureter with high stone clearance rates and limited morbidity.

Box 7.1 Indications for ureteroscopic treatment of calculi

- ESWL failure (including contraindications to ESWL treatment)
- Impacted calculi
- Large stones (>10 mm)
- Multiple stones
- Associated with distal obstruction
- Solitary kidney
- Bilateral ureteric calculi

Indications for the endoscopic treatment of ureteric calculi are provided in Box 7.1. In most centres, ESWL is the preferred treatment option for proximal ureteric calculi and distal ureteric calculi <10 mm; contraindications or ESWL are listed in Box 7.2. Indeed some surgeons prefer to try

ESWL to treat most ureteric stones regardless of site and proceed to ureteroscopy only after failure of ESWL.

Box 7.2 Contraindications to ESWL

- Morbid obesity
- Anticoagulation
- Aortic aneurysm
- Pregnancy

THE SEMIRIGID URETEROSCOPE

In 1962 McGovern and Walzack used a 9F flexible endoscope transurethrally to visualise a distal ureteric stone. The late 1970s witnessed the development of rigid ureteroscopy and in 1981 Das reported the first case of transurethral ureteroscopy with stone basketing under direct vision. In 1988 the smaller and flexible semirigid ureteroscope was introduced. The semirigid ureteroscope has been further developed and remains the main endoscope for ureteroscopic management of ureteric calculi.

Semirigid ureteroscopy is ideal for most procedures whilst the flexible ureterorenoscope is useful for stones in the proximal ureter where access with the semirigid ureteroscope can be difficult. Since the introduction of the 6.9F semirigid ureteroscope only a very small proportion of ureters now require preintubation dilatation. The latest versions of the scopes have two separate working channels predominantly designed to allow a type of continuous-flow, low-pressure irrigation which is particularly valuable during laser lithotripsy.

URETEROSCOPY

The following sequence is considered:
- Pre-operative checklist (Box 7.3)
- Theatre environment/patient positioning
- Ten operative steps (Box 7.4)

Box 7.3 Ureteroscopy: pre-operative checklist

(1) *Serum analyses:* check sodium and creatinine

(2) *Urine:* recent microscopy, cultures and sensitivity should be known

(3) *Consent:* inform the patient of alternatives to treatment and risks of surgery (ureteric perforation, avulsion and stricture formation – see Chapter 11). Tell them of the possibility of stent insertion and need for ancillary procedures if stone left behind

(4) *Pre-operative imaging:* all pre-operative images including a recent KUB should be available in theatre

(5) *Mark:* put an arrow on the lower flank of the correct side with indelible ink

(6) *Radiographer notified:* fluoroscopy has to be available for the entirety of the procedure

(7) *Female patients:* as radiography will be used, confirm the patient is not pregnant

(8) *Antibiotics:* patients should receive one dose of broad-spectrum intravenous antibiotics at induction

(9) *Operating table:* ensure correct table for radiography

(10) *Anticipate technical difficulties:* large prostate, previous pelvic surgery, radiation or trauma

---

Theatre environment/patient positioning

The patient should be placed in the Lloyd-Davies extended lithotomy position (see Chapter 4, Figure 4.2) onto a table suitable for radiography. The theatre environment should be arranged so that equipment and instruments are available to hand at ease, with an uninterrupted line of vision from the seated surgeon to the video monitor and fluoroscopy screen (Figure 4.3, Figure 7.2). The arms and hands of the patient should be secured to the patient's side instead of being folded on the chest, as in the latter position they are often in the way when the kidneys are screened.

> **Box 7.4 Operative steps for ureteroscopy and intracorporeal lithotripsy**
>
> (1) Cystoscopy
> (2) Insertion of safety guidewire
> (3) Ureteric catheter insertion and retrograde ureteropyelography (optional)
> (4) Intubation of ureter with URS and stone access
> (5) Stone fragmentation
> (6) Fragment retrieval
> (7) Flexi URS (optional)
> (8) Retrograde ureterogram (optional)
> (9) Post-treatment renal drainage (stent or catheter) (optional)
> (10) Bladder drainage (optional)

Ureteroscopy: the ten steps

(1) Start with cystoscopy

Perform cystoscopy to exclude calculus in the bladder, to assess the VUJ and to exclude synchronous disease.

(2) Positioning the safety wire in the kidney

Under continuous fluoroscopic control, a safety wire is passed up the ureter into the renal pelvis using the Albaran bridge of the cystoscope. The standard safety wire is a 0.038 inch PTFE straight floppy-tip guidewire.

> **DON'T!** Take care not to dislodge the stone proximally with the guidewire

Guidewire passage past a stone or a tortuous, angled ureter can be difficult. Hydrophilic wires should be turned to as soon as it is seen that the standard wire will not pass the calculus after three gentle attempts. The safety wire should then be left *in situ* until the end of the procedure and is there to allow access to the kidney for ureteric stenting should complications arise during the procedure (Figure 7.3). Second wires introduced via the endoscope can act as working wires.

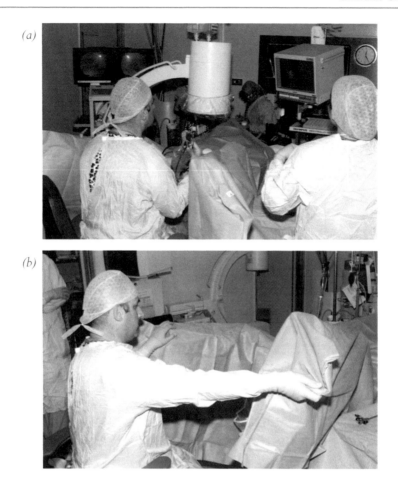

Figure 7.2 (a) Ureterorenoscopy in progress, (b) manipulation of the leg during the procedure can be valuable.

DO! Once a hydrophilic wire is in the renal pelvis exchange it for a standard wire over an open-ended ureteral catheter

The rigidity of the guidewire helps straighten out angles in the ureter and facilitates the introduction of the ureteroscope and insertion of balloon dilators, catheters and stents. It opens up the ureteric orifice and separates the ureteral walls. It also serves to identify the ureteric orifice during multiple insertions of the ureter. The guidewire chosen depends on what is encountered. Not all urologists use safety wires but they are invaluable during training. The old adage applies that one rarely regrets using one but may often regret not using one!

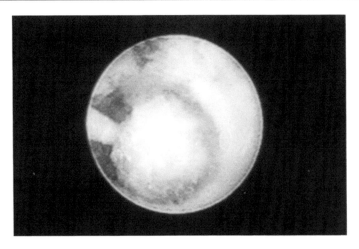

Figure 7.3 Safety wire in situ *alongside calculus in mid ureter.*

(3) Perform a retrograde ureteropyelogram

In cases of diagnostic uncertainty retrograde ureteropyelography can delineate the anatomy and help avoid complications. A size 5 or 6F open-ended ureteric catheter (olive tip) is placed in the ureteric orifice and a small amount of dilute contrast medium (50:50) is injected under low pressure. Continuous fluoroscopy is performed as the contrast is injected and the outline of the ureter visualised to provide the diagnostic information required (Figure 7.4).

> **DO!** Exclude air bubbles from the contrast syringe and flush the catheter before intubation to exclude air bubbles in the ureter being mistaken for calculi

(4) Semirigid ureteroscopy

This is performed alongside the safety wire. The passage through the urethra into the bladder, especially in men through the prostatic urethra, must be done carefully with the lumen in the centre of the screen to avoid false passage formation.

Once in the bladder the ureter is assessed endoscopically and intubated as atraumatically as possible. Inversion of the scope will aid most intubations and if awkward a second wire can be passed and used to open up the ureteric

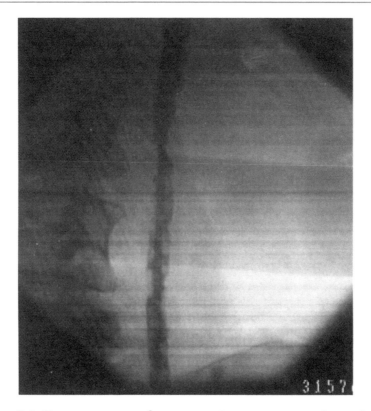

Figure 7.4 Fluoroscopic image after a retrograde ureterogram revealing multiple filling defects throughout the ureter. This patient had ureteritis cystica.

orifice and the scope passed between the two wires ('riding the tracks' – see Chapter 4 on how to overcome a difficult ureteric orifice).

Inside the ureter, the scope should be advanced methodically under continuous vision using the guidewire as a reference point. The lumen should be visible at all times (see Figure 4.8). The mucosa should be seen directly underneath and should pass by smoothly without bunching or telescoping. The irrigation should be kept sufficiently high to allow suitable irrigant flow (Figure 7.5).

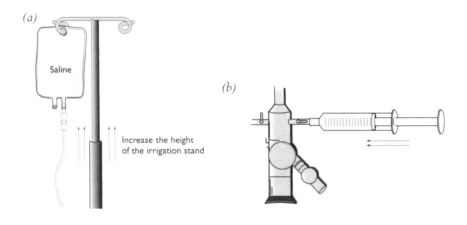

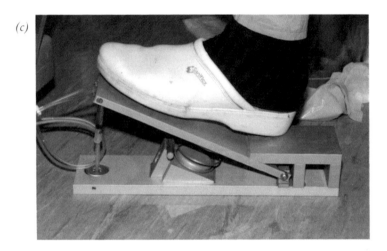

Figure 7.5 Methods for maintaining irrigant flow. (a) Increasing the height of the irrigant fluid bag; (b) Injecting saline through a syringe; (c) Irrigation system allowing continuous irrigation supplemented by aliquots of fluid via the foot-operated syringe (Peditron).

DON'T! Beware of pushing stone fragments backwards with high irrigant flow

(5) Intracorporeal lithotripsy

Small stones can be extracted under vision whilst larger or impacted stones have to be fragmented to less than 2–3 mm in order to pass freely or to be removed. Energy sources available for stone fragmentation include electro-hydraulic, ultrasonic, laser (holmium or pulsed dye) and pneumatic (Lithoclast) devices. The present gold standard is the holmium laser. Table 7.3 lists the various lithotripsy methods available for ureteroscopy.

> DO! If there is too much bleeding or too much debris, aspirate with a 20 ml syringe via the instrument channel or keep the second channel open throughout the procedure

Table 7.3 Lithotripsy methods available for ureteroscopy

Lithotripsy	Advantage	Disadvantage
Ultrasound	Able to aspirate fragments	Large calibre – not suitable for ureteroscopy
Electrohydraulic	Good fragmentation	Can damage urothelium Difficult to control
Laser	Flexible, small fibres Minimal propulsion Very controllable	Expensive Fragile fibres Slow
Ballistic (Lithoclast)	Easy to use Inexpensive Will break most stones Controllable	Propulsion of fragments Will not break all stones

(6) Stone retrieval

Once the calculus has been fragmented it is our practice to retrieve all frag-ments and aim for endoscopic and fluoroscopic stone clearance. Retrieval of fragments can be achieved with a variety of ancillary instruments, but generally triradiate forceps and baskets (Figure 7.6) are in commonest use.

The advantage of forceps is that the stone will be released from the grip of the instrument if some resistance is encountered during withdrawal. Basketing can be dangerous if too large or too many fragments are entrapped

Box 7.5 Basket or triradiate forceps?	
Basket	**Triradiate forceps**
Efficient	Only small volume of stone removed
Quick clearance	Slow
May become impacted	Will not become entrapped

and cannot negotiate narrower segments of the ureter downstream (see Box. 7.5). Figure 7.7 illustrates how to catch a stone with a basket device.

In this situation one must not pull for fear of tearing the ureter or even avulsing it. The calculi will need to be further fragmented in the basket. This can be achieved if the instrument channel will accommodate a laser fibre, but generally there is not enough space. In this situation the balloon handle should be detached and the outer sheath of the basket removed (Figure 7.8). Usually this will then allow sufficient room to accommodate the lithotriptor in the channel and the calculus can be further fragmented *in situ* and basket with or without fragments removed.

If there is still insufficient room, the ureteroscope can be removed over the basket and passed alongside to fragment the stone within the basket, which can be subsequently withdrawn (Figure 7.9).

Retrieval of fragments can be done in stages and this prevents the above complications. Be aware that a fragmented calculus has a larger surface area than an unfragmented stone. Once fragments have been retrieved they can be left in the bladder to be voided later on by the patient.

TIP! Before basket retrieval
- Know how to dismantle the basket before using it
- Know the space available in the instrument channel – will it accommodate the lithotripsy device and a basket?

---

(7) Flexible ureterorenoscopy (flexi URS)

If a stone in the proximal ureter is difficult to reach and treat with the semi-rigid scope or there is stone in the intrarenal collecting system then the flexi URS should be used. Flexible ureterorenoscopy is often a two-man, two-hand job that requires frequent intermittent use of fluoroscopy. The operator needs to be in a position that is comfortable and that affords ergonomic

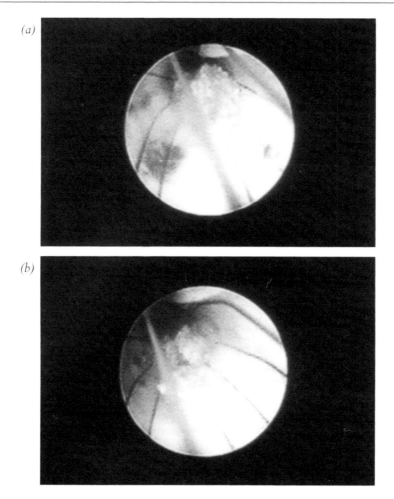

(a)

(b)

Figure 7.6 Basketing. (a) Calculus in basket; (b) following lithotripsy the fragments can be retrieved.

efficiency with no wastage of hand movements. The thumb of the dominant hand should be on the active deflector lever, whilst the other hand stabilises the shaft of the ureteroscope at the urethral meatus (see Figures 7.10 and 7.11).

> **DON'T!** Do not twist the shaft of the flexible scope at the meatus without moving the wrist in the same direction as this movement can damage the fibreoptic bundles

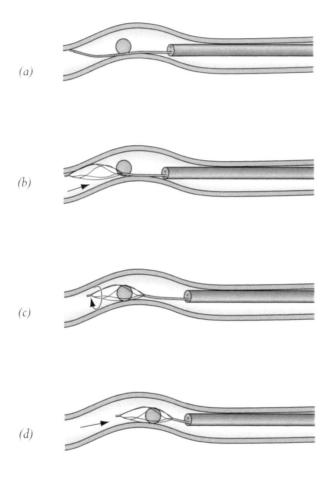

Figure 7.7 *How do you catch a stone with a basket? (a) Pass beyond the stone with endoscopic and fluoroscopic imaging. (b) Open basket, Pull back. (c) Rotate the basket slowly around the stone and engage stone within the basket. Ensure no urothelium is caught in the basket. (d)Withdraw gently.Watch wall of ureter and ensure basket moves in relation to wall. If not, disengage. Do not pull. If there is any resistance, stop.*

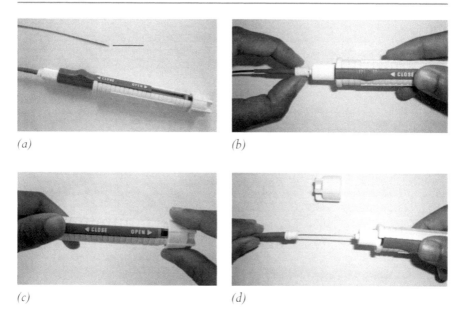

(a)   (b)

(c)   (d)

*Figure 7.8 How do you dismantle the basket handle? (a) Basket in closed position (arrow). (b) Unscrew the luer lock connector at the sheath/handle junction. (c) Unscrew the flange cap at the proximal end of the handle. (d) Slide the handle off of the mandrel. *Photos depict basket handle of Parachute™ (Boston Scientific). Basket devices differ in their assembly – always read the instructions before using it!*

A summary of key points during flexi URS is listed below and the reader is referred to the description of the technique in Chapter 4:

* Rotate the scope so that the working channel and wire are at 12 o'clock, this prevents the tip from hitting the roof of the ureteric orifice when entering.
* Buckling can decrease the amount of active deflection available (Box 7.6).

Box 7.6 How to avoid buckling

* 'Play it straight' – keep the ureteroscope straight from urethral meatus to lens
* In bladder: make sure wire is under tension as it enters the ureteric orifice
* In urethra: for men, the assistant holds the penis at stretch to prevent buckling in the urethra

---

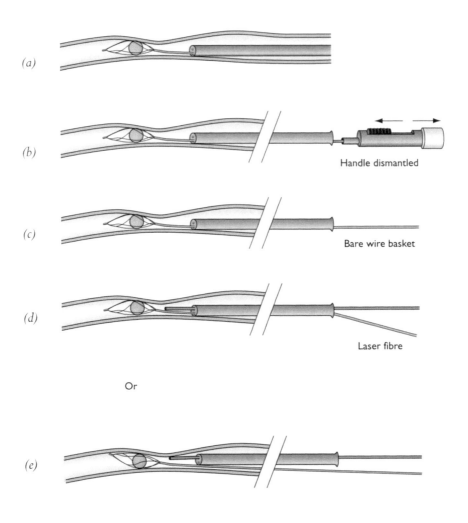

(a)

(b) Handle dismantled

(c) Bare wire basket

(d) Laser fibre

Or

(e)

Figure 7.9 Steps to deal with basket trapped by impacted calculus. (a) Basket closed and trapped by impacted calculus. (b) Dismantle the basket. (c) Bare wire basket now in place (sheath removed). (d) Sufficient room to pass Lithoclast or laser to fragment stone in basket. (e) Ureteroscope taken off basket and reintroduced alongside to fragment stone with laser.

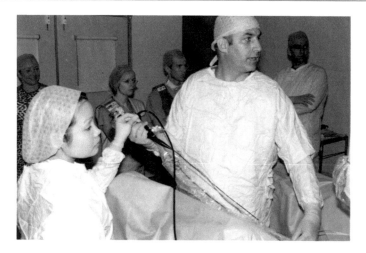

Figure 7.10 Insertion of flexi URS over a Superstiff™ guidewire. Note the passage is being monitored on fluoroscopy and the scope is being passed whilst counter traction is applied by the nurse on the wire ensuring the wire remains in the kidney.

- If the flexi URS will not proceed because of a narrowing in the ureter, a transureteroscopic balloon dilatation device (Passport™, Boston Scientific) can be employed (Figure 7.12).
- Once in the renal calyces, a 365 μm holmium laser fibre in the working channel can be replaced by a 200 μm fibre to allow increased deflection of the scope.

Figure 7.13 shows calculi visualised in the calyx during flexi URS.

(8) Retrograde ureteropyelogram

At the end of the procedure a retrograde ureteropyelogram may be performed to exclude perforation/extravasation and to identify the renal pelvis for subsequent ureteric stent insertion.

(9) Post-treatment renal drainage

Insert a ureteric stent or catheter if required (see below).

(a)

(b)

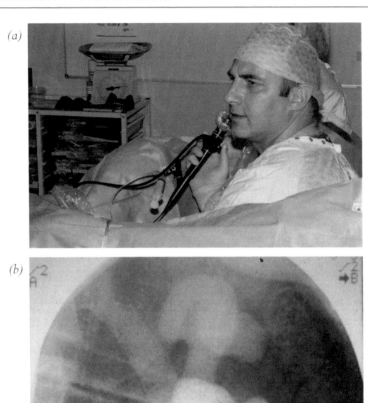

Figure 7.11 (a) Flexi URS in position. The thumb of the dominant hand is activating the deflection lever. Note the three-way tap on irrigation port with contrast filled syringe. (b) Flexi URS in the intrarenal collecting system on fluoroscopy.

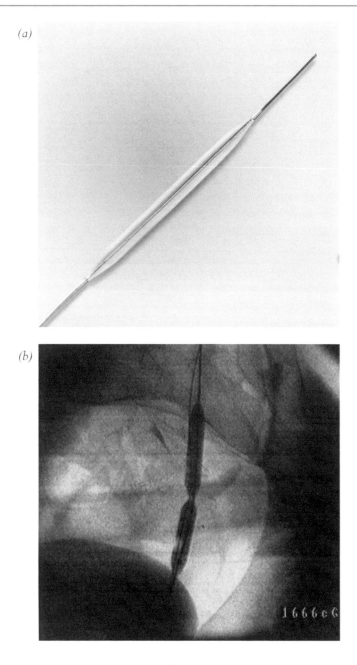

Figure 7.12 Intra-ureteric balloon dilatation. (a) This small balloon on a guidewire (Passport™) can be passed via the instrument channel of the semirigid URS to allow balloon dilatation of the ureter under direct vision and with simultaneous fluoroscopy if required (courtesy of Boston Scientific). (b) Fluoroscopic image demonstrating 'waisting' during balloon dilatation of a ureteric stricture.

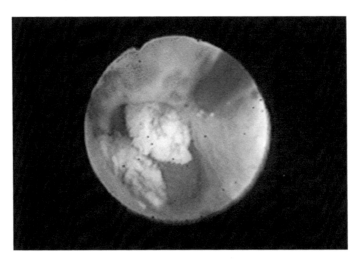

Figure 7.13 Calculi visualised in calyx at flexi URS. Laser fibre visible in the 10 o'clock position prior to intracorporeal laser fragmentation.

(10) Bladder drainage

If the procedure is prolonged, bloody or being performed in an elderly man with an enlarged prostate a post-operative urethral catheter can be placed and removed early the following morning.

> **DO!** Place a urethral catheter if concerned about sepsis to ensure low pressure in renal pelvis for 24–48 hours

OBSTRUCTIVE URETERIC LITHIASIS

In a patient with acute calculus obstruction and infection, ureteroscopic treatment is contraindicated. Fragmentation of calculi in this situation can lead to release of endotoxins from the stone and pyelovenous absorption. Drainage of the upper tract should be achieved either by nephrostomy tube placement or retrograde ureteric stent insertion. Neither method has been shown to be superior (Pearle et al, 1998), although the former avoids a general anaesthetic and can sometimes be technically easier than trying to get a stent passed an impacted ureteric calculus. Ureteroscopy may be performed only after the sepsis has resolved.

> **DON'T!** Endoscopic manipulation of the upper urinary tract in the presence of sepsis and calculus obstruction can exacerbate urosepsis and lead to septicaemia, multi-organ failure and even death

STONE RETRIEVAL AND TRICKS

Stone-free rate and location

The success rate of clearing calculi is dependent on the correct use of the various endoscopes and ancillary equipment available. Larger stone size and a proximal ureteral location are independent predictors of treatment failure (Hollenbeck et al., 2001). The modern-day stone-free rate for treating distal ureteric calculi is above 95% (Tawfiek & Bagley, 1999). This rate is however lower, around 80%, when treating proximal ureteric calculi (Hollenbeck et al., 2001). This is likely to improve as instrumentation and endoscopic skills improve.

Tricks

Box 7.7 lists some tricks that may be tried when the passage of a guidewire is impeded by an impacted stone. The reader should be familiar with how to dismantle a basket device (Figure 7.8) and be able to deal with the basket trapped by impacted calculi (Figure 7.9). Propulsion and proximal migration of calculi is often seen when the Lithoclast® is used to fragment stones. Steps to deal with this problem are given in Box 7.8.

Box 7.7 Tricks to overcome an impacted stone with a guidewire

(1) Inject a small amount of contrast slowly using the ureteral catheter to define the exact ureteric anatomy.
(2) Change the guidewire to a hydrophilic one.
(3) Use a ureteral catheter: open-ended or angled, to stabilise the guidewire.
(4) Use a semirigid scope and pass the guidewire under vision.
(5) Consider breaking the stone carefully then pass the wire when the way through is visualised.
(6) Injection of ureteric lignocaine to reduce spasm.
(7) Consider percutaneous access and antegrade ureteroscopy or laparoscopic ureterolithotomy.

Box 7.8 Tricks to prevent proximal migration of calculi or fragment

- Irrigation is slowed to a trickle
- Basket or holding device deployed (Lithocatch™ or Stone cone™)
- Use laser over Lithoclast®
- Beware hydrostatic pressure may flush the stone (excessive retrograde ureterogram and irrigation)
- Use flexi URS and chase
- Tilt patient's head up
- Stop all irrigation

STENTING

The absolute indication for ureteric stent insertion after ureteroscopy is for a confirmed ureteral perforation. The relative indications for ureteric stent insertion are listed in Table 7.4.

Stent-related symptoms

Ureteric double-pigtail stents can be quite uncomfortable. Up to 80% of patients can experience irritative voiding symptoms. Haematuria, flank and

Table 7.4 Relative indications for stent insertion after ureteroscopy

- Significant ureteral oedema at stone impaction site which can lead to temporary ureteric obstruction
- Impaired renal function
- Solitary kidney
- Transplant kidney
- Recent urinary tract infection or sepsis
- Following ureteral dilatation $+/-$ splitting
- Large residual fragment burden
- Failed ureteroscopy and need to dilate the ureter
- Patient factors (e.g. distance to hospital, pregnancy)
- Initial stone burden >2 cm
- Longstanding impacted stone

suprapubic pain are common stent-related symptoms, and in one study up to 70% of patients needed analgesia for stent-related pain (Joshi et al., 2003). As a result of our understanding of the morbidity of stents, stents are used more judiciously and their use has decreased in recent years.

Altering the material or the size of the stent has been shown to have no impact on stent-related symptoms. A randomised study comparing 4.7F and 6F double-pigtail ureteral stents in patients following ureteroscopy and holmium laser lithotripsy showed no significant differences with respect to irritative voiding symptoms or pain. Instead, smaller stents were associated with significant proximal migration and early removal (Erturk et al., 2003). Tailed stents have been found to cause fewer voiding symptoms than double J stents. However, they may fail to prevent stricture formation at the distal tailed end. Stent placement technique may have an effect on symptoms. Rane et al. (2001) found that stents crossing the mid-line in the bladder and incomplete loops at the distal tail end resulted in more symptoms.

To stent or not to stent?

Miniaturisation of ureteroscopes combined with improvements in intra-corporeal lithotripsy resulting in smaller stone fragments, especially after holmium laser lithotripsy, has reduced the morbidity of ureteroscopy and hence the need for post-procedure stenting.

Stenting after ureteroscopy need not be done if ureteroscopy was uncom-plicated and residual stone fragments are small (<3 mm). Ureteral perforation at the site of the stone is the primary risk factor for stricture formation, and a stent must always be placed in this scenario. It should also be considered when dilatation of the ureter is required in order to avoid possible obstruction from post-procedure oedema.

Stent insertion and tricks

The different types of stents available are detailed in Chapter 3. Getting the length of the stent right is important; excessive length leads to increased irritative symptoms, whilst too short a length increases the risk of migration. Box 7.9 lists aids to choosing the right length. Figure 7.14 goes through the steps required for retrograde stent insertion.

Box 7.9 Choosing the correct stent length

- Sex: choose shorter sizes in women
- Height: one formula is height < 5 ft 10 in: 22 cm long; 5 ft 10 in to 6 ft 4 in: 24 cm; > 6 ft 4 in: 26 cm*
- Ureteric length:
  (1) Measure ureter length on an IVU
  (2) Measure the length of the ureter – place a guidewire into the ureter, gradually pull back till the tip is at the level of the PUJ and make a bend in the wire (or clip on an artery forceps); pull the wire further back till the tip is at the VUJ and make another bend. The distance between the bends is the length of the ureter
* This formula works with normally sited ureters. In the presence of abnormal anatomy (e.g ileostomy and implanted ureters) allowances need to be made

---

DO! Monitor for post-obstructive diuresis after exchange of an obstructed stent

---

DO! It can be difficult to insert a stent over a hydrophilic wire. Exchange it for a working PTFE wire over a 5 or 6F open-ended ureteric catheter

---

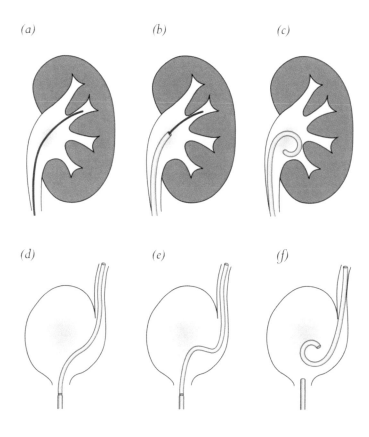

(a)   (b)   (c)

(d)   (e)   (f)

Figure 7.14 Ureteric JJ stent placement. (a) Retrograde pyelogram with wire in renal pelvis. (b) Stent passed over wire (finer tip fed first) and number of markers on stent noted. Pusher fed over wire (marker first) so that the stent passes over the wire into renal pelvis. **DO!** Follow stent progress over the wire on fluoroscopy and endoscopic monitor. **DO!** Push stent through whilst keeping the guidewire straight and under tension. **DO!** Check the guidewire position – make sure your assistant keeps it fixed in place. (c) Wire removed and stent pushed as coil is formed in pelvis. (d) Once upper coil is in pelvis, lower end directed into middle bladder. (e) Once end of stent visualised, wire is removed whilst pushing into middle bladder. (f) Coil formed in bladder. Remove pusher.

> DON'T! When the upper ureter is dilated, make sure the pigtail is in the renal pelvis and not in the ureter itself

> DON'T! When inserting a stent in the presence of a nephrostomy tube ensure they do not coil together!

Assessing ureteral stent patency

No imaging method is fully specific for the diagnosis of ureteric stent obstruction. Routine assessment of stent patency is therefore not cost-effective and most centres simply adhere to a regular stent change policy (every 4–6 months). However, Box 7.10 lists the methods that can help in the evaluation of stent function.

Box 7.10 Evaluating stent function

(1) Grey scale ultrasound – this is very unreliable, as renal dilatation may merely reflect reflux through a patent stent. But new or increased dilatation is very suspicious

(2) Colour Doppler ultrasound – can be used to assess urine flow through the lower pigtail into the bladder. But absent colour signals can also be seen with patent stents

(3) Contrast cystography – to look for reflux up the stent and into the kidney. Said to be 70–80% accurate

(4) Diuretic renogram (MAG 3 or DTPA) – reflux up patent stent makes analysis difficult. About 75% accuracy

---

Management of retained stents/encrusted stents

Stent related complications are listed in Box 7.11. Encrustation is a common problem (Box 7.12). Not all encrusted stents are difficult to remove. Removal of a stuck encrusted stent requires lots of manipulation. This increases the risk of shedding endotoxins from the encrustations upstream, and so adequate antibiotic cover at surgery is necessary. Management requires use of a combination of cystolitholapaxy, URS, ESWL, PCNL and antegrade URS (Figure 7.15).

> DO! If removal of an encrusted stent was difficult, continue antibiotics for a week after surgery

Encrustation may be at the tip (Figure 7.16) or through the whole length of the stent with varying amounts of stone burden in the bladder, ureter and kidney. CT can be helpful in assessing the stone burden (Box 7.13). Calcium oxalate/phosphate followed by struvite are the most common components. If encrustation is marked (linear encrustation >6 mm) try ESWL first. If using the semirigid URS with holmium laser to break up the encrustated stent, we recommend setting at a low power (5 W). The laser beam must be aimed perpendicular to the stone, parallel to the ureter and parallel to the stent. Start at one point until the stent is exposed and then directly treat the calcifications, freeing the calcifications from the stent and then directly breaking the free stones with the laser fibre. Good visibility is the key to success. Beware of breaking a wire or the stent. If retrograde or antegrade methods to remove the stent fail, laparoscopic or open surgery should be considered.

> DO! If the encrusted stent will not allow the URS to pass, leave a 4.7F ureteric stent parallel with the stent and come back after a few weeks as this will allow the ureter to passively dilate further

---

Box 7.11 Complications with stents

- Stent-related symptoms
- Proximal migration
- Distal migration can lead to incontinence
- Incrustation (endoluminal crusts)
- Encrustation (extraluminal crusts)
- Obstruction leading to loss of kidney function
- Fracture
- Urosepsis/urinary tract infections – biofilm formation

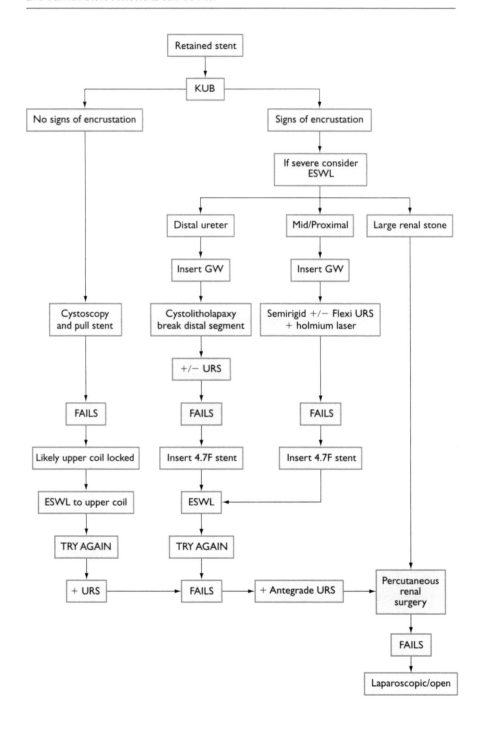

Figure 7.15 Algorithm for the management of the encrusted stent.

Box 7.12 Risk factors for encrustation

* Long indwelling time
* History of stone disease
* Chemotherapy
* Pregnancy
* Severe UTI and concurrent sepsis
* Renal impairment
* Anatomical and metabolic abnormalities

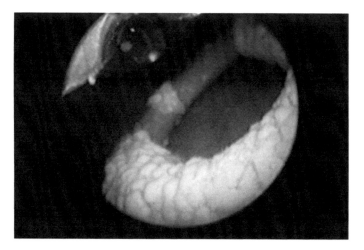

Figure 7.16 Endoscopic view of encrustation around the distal coil of a ureteric stent that had been left in place for 7 months.

Management of proximally migrated stent

Proximal migration may occur when the stent is too short for the ureter. The incidence of stent migration is 2–4%. Retrieval should be done under direct vision using the ureteroscope and triradiate graspers or basket to catch the stent and pull it down. Balloon dilators have been used under screening to retrieve stents, but we feel this method is not as effective, and dilates the ureter causing further proximal migration.

DO! If exchanging a migrated stent, replace with a longer stent

---

Box 7.13 Telling stent from stone on CT

Using the bone window setting on CT, stents can be visually distinguished from calculi. Stents are denser than calculi and have a Hounsfield unit range between 1600 and 2600

Stent removal

Up to 40–50% of stents may become encrusted at 12 weeks, so try to remove all stents by 3 months. It is the responsibility of the physician inserting the stent to ensure follow-up and removal. The importance of maintaining an adequate recall system, such as a computerised record, along with informing patients about the hazards of a retained stent cannot be overstressed. The forgotten ureteric stent can be a disastrous complication for the patient, with litigious consequences for the surgeon.

POST-URETEROSCOPY CARE

Most patients can be discharged on resumption of voiding. Following ureteroscopy, patients can expect to feel intermittent flank pain, dysuria and haematuria. In our experience, patients informed of these symptoms before surgery are able to cope with them better post-operatively. Daycase ureteroscopy is now commonplace, but complex ureterorenoscopy may require inpatient admission for management of the catheter, sepsis and pain (Box 7.14).

Box 7.14 Criteria for inpatient admission following ureteroscopy

---

(1) Fever
(2) Unduly long procedure with excess instrumentation
(3) Suspicion of ureteral perforation
(4) Heavy bleeding
(5) Pain not controlled with oral analgesia
(6) Social factors – patient lives too far from an emergency department

---

Patient advice

Fluid intake should be increased for the first couple of days to ensure a good diuresis to prevent any possible clot formation. Fifty per cent of patients can be back to work within 4 days, whilst nearly all patients will be at work and full exercise within 2 weeks. They should be advised to attend the emergency department if they suffer intractable pain, persistent nausea and vomiting, high fever, severe frank haematuria or urinary retention.

Immediate post-operative care

In the immediate post-operative period, the main things to watch out for are sepsis and upper tract obstruction. The chance of urosepsis after manipulation of the upper tract is higher in the presence of a positive urine culture, and these patients would benefit from further doses of antibiotics, as should patients who have a recognised ureteral perforation and indwelling ureteral stent in place. Stent-related symptoms may respond to antimuscarinics and oral analgesics. Obstruction of the upper tract can present as intractable pain and may be a result of retained fragments, clot obstruction, sepsis or, if a stent is used, stent migration leading to obstruction.

Long-term problems

The incidence of stricture formation following ureteroscopy and stenting is 1%, but this is higher if there has been an intraoperative perforation. Most strictures present within the first 6 months. Patients at risk of stricture formation should get an IVU or ultrasound within 2–3 weeks, with a repeat at 3 months to rule out silent obstruction. Sometimes stone fragmentation expels stones into the retroperitoneum, recognised at ureteroscopy. In these circumstances the patient should be informed of the fragments' location on radiography, in order to avoid confusion in the future.

Retained fragments

In the situation where stone clearance has not been possible it is sensible to stent the ureter and for the patient to return a few weeks later. The calculi and stent can be removed remarkably easy with limited constitutional upset for the patient.

DIFFICULT CASES: PREGNANCY AND THE URETERIC STONE

Ureteric colic during pregnancy requires accurate imaging and confident and reliable urological input. Delays in diagnosis and treatment can lead to premature labour and prolonged unnecessary maternal suffering. The most important aspect of managing this situation is establishing a diagnosis. The investigation of choice is an urgent MRI, which has no proven toxicity for the baby or the mother. If this is not available, and ultrasound has not added useful diagnostic information and the diagnosis is in doubt, a limited IVU should be performed. This should identify the location and size of the obstructing calculus.

Currently, ureteroscopy and stone clearance during pregnancy is probably the treatment of choice, although many still favour a conservative approach. Experience has taught us that the ureteroscopy may be surprisingly easy and not as limited by the gravid uterus as expected. Stone clearance rates can be excellent and it is a most satisfying procedure to perform. Clearly fluoroscopic exposure to the fetus must be kept to a minimum, but delays in diagnosis and mismanagement of ureteric colic during pregnancy can have devastating results.

REFERENCES

Das S. Transurethral ureteroscopy and stone manipulation under direct vision. J Urol 1981; 125: 112–3

Erturk E, Sessions A, Joseph JV. Impact of ureteral stent diameter on symptoms and tolerability. J Endourol 2003; 17: 59–62

Hollenbeck BK, Schuster TG, Faerber GJ, Wolf JS Jr. Comparison of outcomes of ureteroscopy for ureteral calculi located above and below the pelvic brim. Urology 2001; 58: 351–6

Joshi HB, Stainthorpe A, MacDonagh RP, et al. Indwelling ureteral stents: evaluation of symptoms, quality of life and utility. J Urol 2003; 169: 1065–9

Lotan Y, Gettman MT, Roehrborn CG, et al. Management of ureteral calculi: a cost comparison and decision making analysis. J Urol 2002; 167: 1621–9

Pearle MS, Pierce HL, Miller GL, et al. Optimal method of urgent decompression of the collection system for obstruction and infection due to ureteural calculi. J Urol 1998; 160: 1260–4

Rane A, Saleemi A, Cahill D, et al. Have stent-related symptoms anything to do with placement technique? J Endourol 2001; 15: 741–5

Sandhu C, Anson KM, Patel U. Urinary tract stones – part II: current status of treatment. Clin Radiol 2003; 58: 422–33

Tawfiek ER, Bagley DH. Management of upper urinary tract calculi with ureteroscopic techniques. Urology 1999; 53: 25–31

SUGGESTED FURTHER READING

Evans HJ, Wollin TA. The management of urinary calculi in pregnancy. Curr Opin Urol 2001; 11: 379–84

Gettman MT, Segura JW. Management of ureteric stones: issues and controversies. BJU Int 2005; 95 (Suppl 2): 85–93

Knudsen BE, Beiko DT, Denstedt JD. Stenting after ureteroscopy: pros and cons. Urol Clin North Am 2004; 31: 173–80

Lam JS, Gupta M. Tips and tricks for the management of retained ureteral stents. J Endourol 2002; 16: 733–41

Segura, JW, Preminger GM, Assimos DG, et al. Ureteral stones clinical guidelines panel summary report on the management of ureteral calculi. J Urol 1997; 158: 1915–21

8. Renal Calculi (Percutaneous Nephrolithotomy)

Percutaneous nephrolithotomy (PCNL) has now replaced open surgery for removing complex renal stones. Extraction of renal calculi through nephrostomy tracts, placed percutaneously in the presence of an obstructed system or at the time of open surgery, was reported in the early 1970s. However, it was not until 1976 that Fernstrom and Johansson reported the first PCNL, where a percutaneous nephrostomy tract was created specifically for elective percutaneous stone removal (Fernstrom & Johansson, 1976). Modern-day single-stage PCNL has come a long way from this groundbreaking report where PCNL took place over several stages and tract dilatation took anywhere up to 20 days!

At the present time, PCNL is indicated for all renal stones >2 cm and lower pole calculi >1 cm. In addition, it is indicated in cases of abnormal anatomy, ESWL or flexible URS failures. Although the morbidity and hospital stay of patients undergoing PCNL may be higher than other less invasive approaches, this is balanced by greater stone clearance rates.

INDICATIONS FOR PCNL

The indications for PCNL in 2005 are listed in Table 8.1. Recent evidence has demonstrated that PCNL has a greater success rate at clearing lower pole stones compared to ESWL and flexible URS. PCNL has a significantly better 3-month stone-free rate for treating lower pole stones >1 cm compared with ESWL (Albala et al., 2001) and for lower pole stones between 1 and 2.5 cm compared with flexible URS (Kuo et al., 2003).

Relative contraindications include any co-morbid condition that limits general anaesthesia in the prone position (e.g. pulmonary disorders such as obstructive sleep apnoea or obesity) or makes access unsafe (e.g. gross organomegaly). Irreversible coagulopathy and pregnancy are further contra-indications.

Table 8.1 Indications for PCNL

- Any renal stone >2 cm
- Staghorn calculus (Figure 8.1)
- Lower pole stones >1 cm
- Abnormal anatomy: horseshoe kidney, calyceal diverticulum, kyphoscoliosis
- ESWL failure or contraindication
- Hard stones: calcium oxalate monohydrate, cystine calculi
- Stones associated with obstruction: infundibular narrowing, ureteral or PUJ obstruction
- Stones associated with a foreign body
- Failure of conventional treatment

For bilateral renal stone disease requiring PCNL, surgery should be performed on the side of clinical importance first (either symptomatic, infected or obstructed). If no clinical difference exists between the two sides, the better functioning kidney is treated first. This can be done either as a synchronous or a two-staged procedure, depending on surgeon preference.

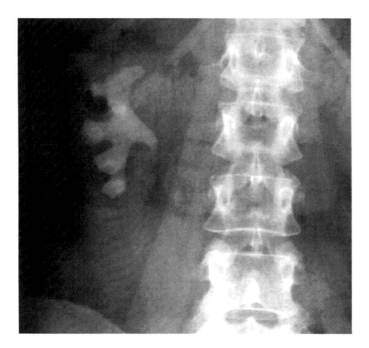

Figure 8.1 A KUB image showing a complete right staghorn calculus.

OPERATIVE TECHNIQUE OF PCNL

PCNL consists of four operative stages: cystoscopy and retrograde ureteral access, percutaneous renal access, tract dilatation and endoscopic stone fragmentation and extraction (Box 8.1). The pre-operative checklist is shown in Box 8.2.

Box 8.1 PCNL: summary of operative steps

---

(1) Ureteric and urethral catheterisation (supine)
(2) Prone positioning of patient
(3) Percutaneous renal access
(4) Tract dilatation
(5) Endoscopic stone fragmentation and extraction (rigid $+-$ flexible endoscopy)
(6) Post-extraction drainage (nephrostomy, ureteric catheter or tubeless)
(7) Wound dressing and care

CYSTOSCOPY AND URETERIC CATHETERISATION

The purpose of cystoscopy is to obtain retrograde ureteric access with a ureteric catheter to allow opacification of the collecting system for percutaneous renal puncture. Ureteric catheterisation holds certain advantages and we always perform this step (Box 8.3). Sometimes retrograde access may be omitted to reduce operative time if a direct puncture onto a stone-bearing calyx is planned.

Procedure

This is performed with the patient supine. Insertion of the ureteric catheter using flexible cystoscopy is technically more difficult than using rigid cystoscopy, but avoids the need for positioning the patient into lithotomy and is our routine. A 6F ureteric catheter with a single end-hole is passed over a standard guidewire into the renal pelvis. A Foley urethral catheter is passed alongside the ureteric catheter whilst holding the latter at the urethral meatus to prevent migration as the Foley catheter is passed. The Foley balloon is inflated and pulled back to the bladder neck. The ureteric catheter is

Box 8.2 PCNL: pre-operative checklist

(1) *Serum analyses:* Hb, platelets, sodium, creatinine, and coagulation screen

(2) *Urine:* recent and previous urine microscopy, cultures and sensitivity must be known

(3) *Drugs:* aspirin, antiplatelet agents and NSAIDS are stopped a week prior to surgery

(4) *Imaging:* IVU is the bare minimum for planning. All pre-operative images including a recent KUB should be available in theatre. Renography should be considered prior to PCNL for staghorn calculi

(5) *Consent:* inform the patient of alternatives to treatment and risks of surgery

(6) *Mark:* put an arrow on the lower flank of the correct side with indelible ink

(7) *Antibiotics:* patients with struvite stones should be given culture-specific antibiotics for 2 weeks prior to PCNL. All patients should receive intravenous antibiotics intra-operatively; we administer a single dose of broad spectrum antibiotics at induction (gentamicin and augmentin)

(8) *Radiographer notified:* image intensifier has to be available for the entirety of the procedure

(9) *Interventional radiologist:* available if required

(10) *Equipment:* radiography table, energy sources, lithotripsy and endoscopes available and working

Box 8.3 Advantages of ureteric catheterisation

- Opacifies and distends the collecting system with contrast agent or air/CO_2 for percutaneous puncture
- Helps identify PUJ during endoscopy; the catheter is seen coming into the renal pelvis
- Limits antegrade passage of stone fragments during stone fragmentation; flushes ureteric calculi into the pelvis

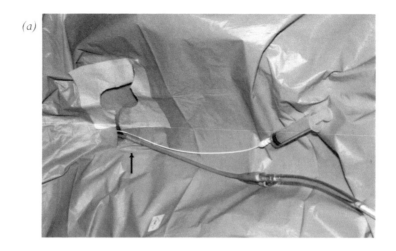

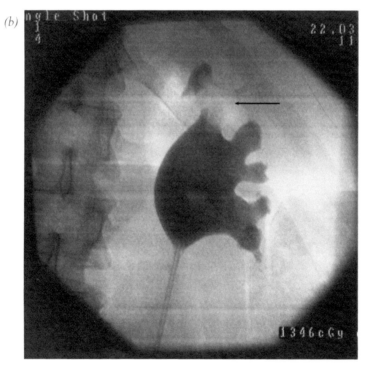

Figure 8.2 Ureteric catheterisation. (a) The ureteric catheter is connected to a syringe and taped to the Foley catheter (arrow). (b) Retrograde ureteropyelogram via ureteric catheter in the prone position with air (arrow) to highlight a posterior calyx for puncture.

positioned as required and taped to the urethral catheter to prevent migration. A 20 ml empty sterile syringe is attached to the end of the ureteric catheter via a Luer connector (Figure 8.2).

PERCUTANEOUS ACCESS

Prone-oblique positioning and draping

PCNL in the supine position is rarely performed. The theatre set-up for PCNL is illustrated in Figure 8.3. Patient positioning to prone-oblique should be done carefully with the anaesthetist co-ordinating events to avoid endotracheal tube dislodgement or injury to the neck or limbs (Figure 8.4). We routinely open the renal angle by rotating the upper torso away from the long axis and lower limbs. In addition, a litre of saline is positioned under the patient in the ipsilateral hypochondrium to provide resistance to kidney migration during tract dilatation (Figure 8.5).

After the skin has been disinfected with an antiseptic solution, a bear-hugger warming blanket is placed over the patient to avoid core temperature fluctuation during the operation (Figure 8.5b). The patient is covered with a waterproof disposable adhesive plastic drape with a see-through window that is placed over the ipsilateral flank. The drape should have a plastic side pouch for collection of irrigation fluid and blood, which is connected to a bucket or a suction device. A rolled up incopad is placed under the medial aspect of the drape to act as a buttress against fluid egress (Figure 8.6).

Sterile drapes must be put on both arms of the C-arm. A giving set is attached via a hole in the drape onto the ureteric catheter (Figure 8.5c).

Access

Percutaneous access is usually obtained in theatre either by the urologist or interventional radiologist. A recent US survey showed that only 11% of urologists obtained their own percutaneous access (Bird et al., 2003). Fluoroscopy and ultrasound are imaging methods commonly employed for gaining access.

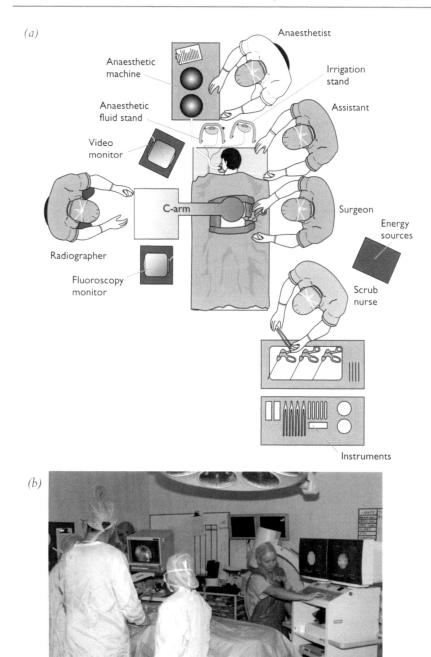

Figure 8.3 (a) Schematic diagram of theatre set-up for PCNL. (b) Theatre set-up for endoscopic stage. Note the C-arm has been withdrawn from the operating field.

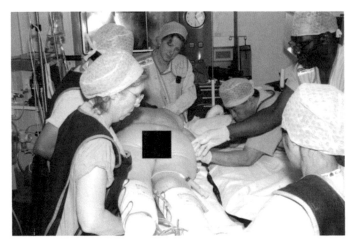

Figure 8.4 Changing patient position from supine to prone-oblique.

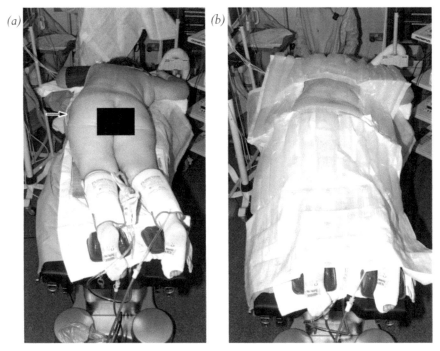

(a)

(b)

Figure 8.5

Figure 8.5 Series of images demonstrating prone-oblique patient positioning. (a) Note: ipsilateral elevation of patient with sandbag (arrow); curved position of patient; head turned to side of stone; attention to arms and padding – pneumatic compression applied to calves; padded donuts at ankle to prevent neuropraxia; image intensifier, endoscopic stack and monitor positioned on side of stone when patient supine. (b) Bear-hugger warming blanket with window over operating site. (c) Patient draped, demonstrating position for fluoroscopy. Intravenous drip extension and syringe connected to ureteral catheter (arrow) for retrograde injection of contrast / air.

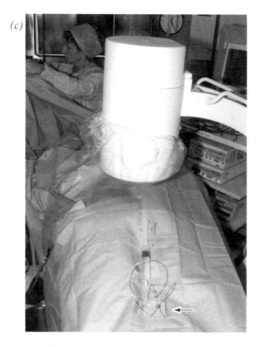

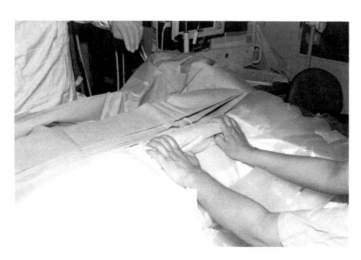

Figure 8.6 Incopad being rolled to prevent fluid egress during surgery.

Puncture

The 12th rib and the posterior mid-axillary line are important anatomical landmarks that help identify the limit of the pleural reflections (see Chapter 5, Figure 5.3). Details of puncture and dilatation are given in Chapter 5, whilst complications of percutaneous access are discussed in Chapter 11.

> DO! Inject air slowly watching constantly under fluoroscopy, to follow the bubbles into the posterior calyces. Remember that air is compressible and gentle injection pressure is best

> DON'T! The right side of the heart is at a lower level than the collecting system in the prone position. Rapid injection of too much air can cause an air embolism. Inject <20 ml slowly, or better still use CO_2. STOP if there is any suggestion of vascular injection or extravasation

Selection of appropriate calyx for access

Understanding the anatomy of the intrarenal collecting system and its relationship to the stone is crucial for successful percutaneous access and retrieval of calculi. The pre-operative images must be studied carefully and a suitable calyx for access should be selected with the likely intraoperative route planned out. Typically the IVU is used for pre-operative planning. The limitation of an IVU is that it is a two-dimensional image of a complex three-dimensional structure, and supplemental information is necessary during fluoroscopy using the rotatable C-arm. Three-dimensional image reconstruction of the pelvi-calyceal system using multislice CT urography is now feasible and can be helpful in the presence of complex anatomy.

A puncture along the axis of the calyx through the papilla has a reduced risk of bleeding. Infundibular punctures are associated with greater risk of bleeding and perforation of the collecting system. Puncture into the pelvis must be avoided due to risk of injury to the posterior branch of the renal artery. These simple technical points that improve the safety margin and success rate of PCNL are further explained in Chapter 5.

Which calyx to target?

The choice of the calyx of entry should be discussed once adequate anatomical information has been obtained from the IVU and fluoroscopy (Figure 8.7). The general considerations at this point are listed in Box 8.4. Anterior calyceal punctures should be avoided, due to possible injury to the arcuate or lobar artery. Mucosal tearing is also more likely as navigation requires the application of considerable torque forces. The posterior calyx is a balance between the least traumatic route into the collecting system and the most direct access to the stone. If the stone lies in a solitary calyx (even if anterior), puncture directly onto a stone-bearing calyx is possible. The relative advantages and de-merits of upper and lower pole calyceal access are compared in Table 8.2.

Box 8.4 General considerations when selecting the calyx to puncture. Also refer to figure 5.14

(1) Complete or maximal stone clearance should be achievable
(2) If complete stone clearance is not possible

- Clear renal pelvis to improve renal drainage
- Clear lower pole calyces as these may not respond to ESWL (residual stones in the upper/interpolar calyces can be treated with ESWL)

(3) Posterior calyces are preferable
(4) Upper pole entry allows access to the PUJ/upper ureter but

- May puncture posterior division artery
- May puncture pleura

DO!
- Keep the axis of the puncture in line with infundibulum
- Keep the long axis of the endoscope in line with the infundibulum during endoscopy to avoid undue torque and trauma to the parenchyma and collecting system

---

Once the appropriate calyx is localised on imaging, a sheath needle (18G translumbar angiography needle) is used to enter the calyx. If it is in the right

(a)

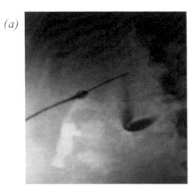

(b)

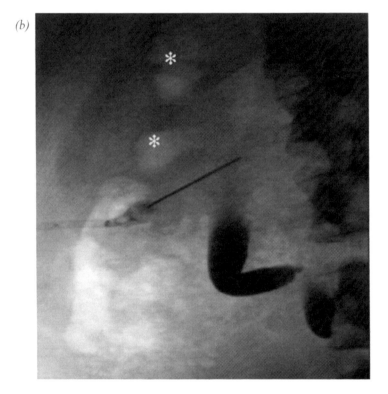

Figure 8.7 (a) and (b) This montage demonstrates the value of double-contrast pyelography for identifying posterior calyces. The patient is in the prone position. In the first image a needle has been inserted under ultrasound guidance and iodinated contrast injected. Being heavier than urine, this has gravitated into the most dependent structure (the ureter). In the second image air/CO_2 has been injected and, being lighter, has gravitated into the least dependent structures, i.e. the posterior facing calyces (starred).

place, urine should be easily aspirated. A guidewire is ideally placed across the PUJ into the bladder to act as a safety wire to allow re-entry should the sheath be dislodged. A hydrophilic guidewire like the Glidewire™ should be used first and positioned in the ureter.

Tract dilatation

Once the calyx is accessed and a guidewire is secured, dilatation progresses as described in Chapters 3 and 5. The use of a stiff guidewire (Amplatz super stiff™, Boston Scientific or Lunderquist, Cook Urological) aids dilatation as its stiffness reorientates the kidney and straightens the lie between the calyx and skin and resists kinking. Tracts can be dilated with either metal telescopic, plastic or balloon dilators (the technical details of these devices and their use are covered in Chapters 3 and 5). Balloon dilatation is quicker and perhaps less traumatic. Retrospective studies have shown balloon dilatation has a lower transfusion rate compared to Amplatz dilators (Davidoff & Bellman, 1997). However the balloon has a tapered tip compared to Amplatz dilators and so it is not easy to use where the stone fills the calyx. Metal dilators are preferred in the obese patient or when there is pre-existing scarring or tight fascia.

Working sheaths

Nephroscopy may be performed without a working sheath, in which case the tract can be smaller. This high-pressure system provides better distension of the collecting system. However, it is not an ideal method because of extravasation and the risk of circulatory overload and sepsis due to excess fluid absorption. Instead, it is usual practice to place a working sheath in the dilated tract through which the nephroscope is inserted.

Low-pressure system

The Amplatz sheath is the most widely used working sheath (Figure 8.8 and Box 8.6). Made of Teflon, it is malleable and has low friction properties. Its length varies from 15 to 20 cm. It can be up to 30F wide. It has an oblique bevelled leading edge, which is 'screwed' into position under fluoroscopy. With the Amplatz, high intrarenal pressures are avoided because irrigant fluid, stone particles and blood clot escape through the space between the sheath and the scope. This means that a drape with a collection and suction device is required to catch all effluxed material.

Table 8.2 Upper pole vs lower pole access

Access	What can you clear?	Advantages	Disadvantages
Lower pole	Most of • lower pole • pelvis • upper pole • interpolar if amenable	• Safe • Posterolateral punctures avoid haemorrhage by going through Brodel's avascular plane • Good visibility	• Parallel lie lower pole calyx unobtainable • PUJ often not easily accessible • Cannot get into mid-pole and PUJ/upper ureter may be difficult
Upper pole	• upper pole, • pelvis • PUJ • lower pole • upper ureter	• Better for obese patients • Good access to pelvis, PUJ and complex lower poles	• Posterior segmental artery injury • If intercostal, increase in morbidity, pleura/parenchymal damage (Box 8.5) • Painful post-operative recovery

TIP!
- For an infra-12th rib upper pole puncture get the anaesthetist to hold the patient's respiration in maximal inspiration. This manoeuvre brings the kidneys away from the pleura (it is pushed away from the 12th rib) and reduces the incidence of thoracic complication
- For a supra 12th rib puncture, hold in maximal expiration as the pleura/lungs are pushed upperwards (but the kidney may also move more cephalad)

DO! Always get a CXR after intercostal punctures. Better still, screen the chest in theatre at the end to reveal any large hydro/pneumothorax. It is easier to insert a chest drain in theatre rather than on the ward

Box 8.5 Complications associated with intercostal punctures

- Pneumothorax and hydrothorax
- Post-operative pain
- Neuralgic pain (nephrostomy tube against periosteum or intercostal nerves)
- Dislodged post-operative drainage tubes

DO! A guidewire must always be in place to maintain access to the collecting system in the unlikely event of sheath withdrawal

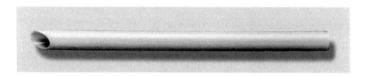

Figure 8.8 The Amplatz sheath (courtesy of Boston Scientific).

Box 8.6 The Amplatz sheath

- Provides access for endoscopic equipment
- Made of PTFE – low friction coefficient and malleable (less likely to buckle)
- Standard size has inner diameter of 30F (able to extract stones <1 cm)
- Bevelled tip can be rotated towards the stone to encourage it into the sheath
- Allows continuous irrigation and low pressure within pelvicalyceal system
- Allows fragments and blood to flush out alongside endoscope

DON'T! The Amplatz sheath, unlike telescoped dilators, does not have a safety stop mechanism. Insertion of these sheaths over coaxial dilators must be done with intermittent screening to avoid pelvic perforation. **DON'T!** push them too far

High-pressure system

Instead of the Amplatz a rigid metallic nephroscope sheath may be used. This is smaller (26F) and permits suction of fluid in the collecting system through a side-arm connection. Constant irrigant flow through the nephroscope with suction through its side-arm creates a continuous-circulation high-pressure system. Figure 8.9 illustrates both low- and high-pressure systems.

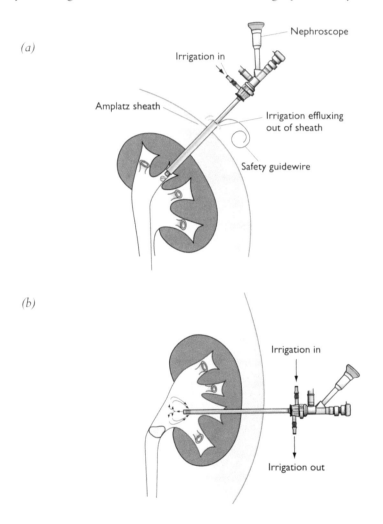

Figure 8.9 Low- and high-pressure irrigation systems used during PCNL. (a) Low-pressure system; (b) High-pressure system.

Loss of working sheath

> **TIP!** Maintain an awareness of the length of the sheath protruding out-
> side the body. If this increases the sheath may have withdrawn. Excessive
> bleeding is another sign of withdrawal. If the track is long, attach an
> artery clip to the tip of the sheath to avoid losing it into the track. If mis-
> placed, carefully replace using the nephroscope as the guide. If this is not
> possible, replace the Amplatz or balloon dilator and replace the sheath

ENDOSCOPIC STONE FRAGMENTATION AND EXTRACTION

Instrumentation

Prior to obtaining percutaneous access, all instrumentation for endoscopy
and stone extraction must be checked (Figure 8.10). The nephroscope, light
source, irrigation and suction equipment must be in working order or you
may find yourself in the precarious position of trying to do an operation with
faulty equipment. It is good practice to have a spare nephroscope available in
case a fault occurs with the one in use during the operation.

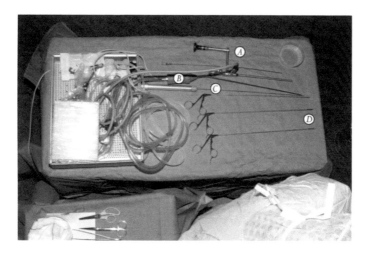

Figure 8.10 Percutaneous renoscopy instrument tray ready for use.
(A) Right angled rigid nephroscope (B) US Lithotripsy (C) Lithoclast® (D) Rigid forceps

> **DO!** Endoscopy is a two-man job. The assistant holds the working sheath/guidewire complex in place, whilst the operator navigates or reinserts the endoscope

Rigid nephroscopy

The rigid nephroscope is the workhorse of PCNL and is preferable to flexible endoscopy due to its better optics, larger irrigation and working channels, superior strength and handling abilities. Nephroscope sizes range from 15 to 26F (see Chapter 3). With rigid nephroscopy, inspection of the pelvis and most calyces should be possible. Care must be taken not to cause mucosal damage/perforation or bleeding.

> **DO!** Use soft wrists and let the anatomy guide the scope rather than the other way around

If the sheath is in the collecting system, the first thing encountered when inserting the nephroscope is usually a blood clot. Clots in the pelvis may be evacuated using forceps (alligator). Adequate irrigation is the key to avoiding future clot formation (Box 8.7). If fat is seen, then the sheath is in the perinephric tissue (either too superficial or too deep through the renal pelvis). Often the target calculus is lying behind or within a clot.

> **DO!** Too much blood? Stop the procedure. Place a large bore drainage tube. Come back 48–72 hours later

---

Box 8.7 Ensuring adequate irrigation

- Enough urine (adequate i.v. fluids administered by anaesthetist)
- Enough warmed isotonic saline irrigation solution
- Always ensure irrigation bag does not run out, especially during 'bloody' procedures
- Keep stand at height 80 cm or less above patient

Flexible nephroscopy

A flexible cystoscope must always be available for PCNL. Inserted through the working sheath, the flexible endoscope allows access to awkward lying infundibula and calyces. At the end of the procedure, all the calyces should be inspected to rule out any retained stone fragments.

Lithrotripsy

Stones <10 mm can be removed intact through a 30F Amplatz sheath (Figure 8.11). Larger stones have to be fragmented with one of the intra-corporeal lithotripsy methods available (see Chapter 3). The pneumatic Lithoclast[®] and ultrasound (US) lithotriptor are the most commonly used devices. US lithotripsy (USL) is particularly valuable for soft 'infection' stones. The Lithoclast[®] is the quickest and most effective for breaking stones, albeit into large fragments (Figure 8.12 and Box 8.8). USL has concomitant suction and is useful for mopping up stones disintegrated into smaller fragments by the Lithoclast[®] (Box 8.9). Likewise, USL can erode stones to a size small enough for grasping with instruments. The combination of USL and the Lithoclast[®] is even more efficient (Swiss Lithoclast Master[®]) and can reduce operative times in comparison with the single energy sources. Holmium laser is ideal for use with the flexible endoscope, although it has a much slower fragmentation rate and is expensive.

Box 8.8 How to break a stone with the Lithoclast[®]

DO! Start in the middle of the calculus and use single pulses	**DON'T!** Multiple pulses at the edge of a stone lead to multiple small fragments that are difficult to clear
DO! Follow fracture lines	
DO! Try to sculpt into large fragments for removal	**DON'T!** Push calculi and fragments too hard – can cause urothelial trauma and bleeding
DO! If stone resistant to single pulse, use multiple pulses	
DO! Watch the whole stone during fragmentation and keep an eye on all pieces	

(a)

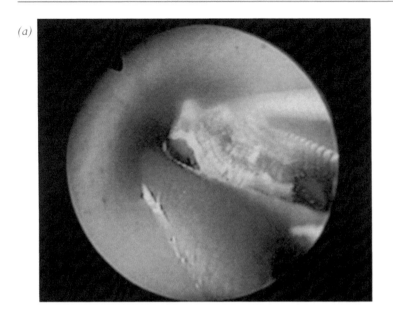

(b)

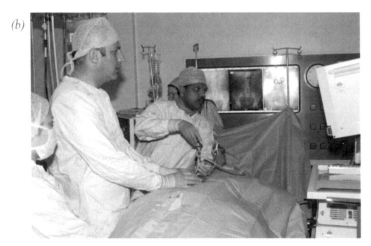

(c)

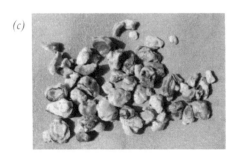

Figure 8.11 (a) Stone fragment being
retrieved with forceps through the
Amplatz sheath during PCNL.
(b) Renoscopy in progress. Note the
assistant keeps control of the Amplatz
sheath and guidewire to prevent
inadvertent loss of access, particularly
during stone retrieval. This patient had
a staghorn calculus fragmented and
removed (c).

(a)

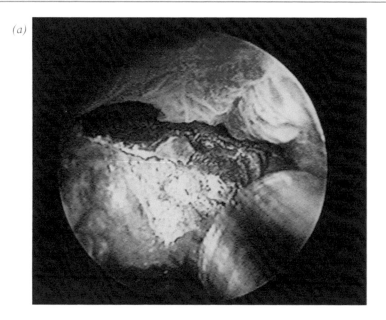

(b)

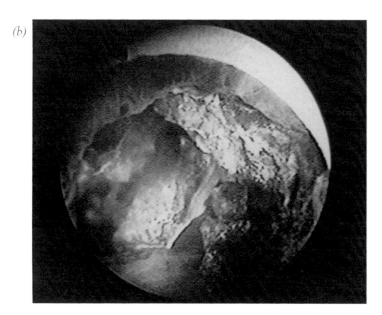

Figure 8.12 (a) and (b) Breaking up the stone during PCNL with the Lithoclast®.

> **Box 8.9 How to break a stone with USL**
>
> | DO! Work on the edge of the calculus
DO! Avoid touching mucosa as it easily bleeds | DON'T! Beware sucking out centre of the stone and leaving an outer shell behind |
> | --- | --- |

> DO! During fragmentation try to track the position of all fragments

Extraction

Stone extraction should always be under direct vision. Equipment available for retrieval includes rigid forceps and disposable baskets and graspers. The alligator forceps are best for grasping small and large fragments (see Chapter 3). When retrieving large fragments use a loose grip when pulling the calculus into the Amplatz sheath. This will often allow the calculus to rotate slowly and be orientated by the edge of the sheath into its longest axis. Once this has been achieved a firmer grip can be applied and the grabbers rotated to ensure the stone can be retrieved safely and not become impacted in the Amplatz.

Baskets are helpful for retrieving fragments that have gone down the upper ureter or into calyces beyond the reach of the endoscope. Nitinol 'tipless' baskets are very useful for fragments in calyces. During flexible nephroscopy stones can be removed using triradiate forceps, baskets or grasping forceps.

> DO! At the end of stone retrieval, the kidney should be screened for any residual fragments

If a stone is found on screening but cannot be immediately located it may be in one of a number of places (Figure 8.14). Once all fragments have been removed an antegrade pyelogram should confirm clearance and the integrity of the collecting system (Figure 8.15).

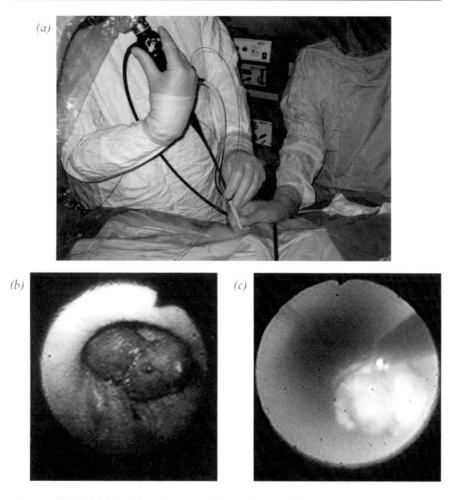

Figure 8.13 *(a) Flexible nephroscopy during PCNL. (b) Calyceal calculi seen at flexible nephroscopy. (c) Basket retrieval of calyceal fragment using the flexible nephroscope.*

STONE CLEARANCE AND HOW TO ACHIEVE IT

The factors that limit complete stone clearance are mainly the limitations imposed by the pelvi-calyceal anatomy. Current nephroscopes are rigid 20–24F instruments, and hence endoscopic navigation of the entire system is often not possible with a single puncture. Flexible nephroscopy allows the rest of the system to be inspected.

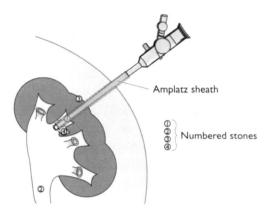

Figure 8.14 Can't find the stone? (1) Behind the sheath? Manipulate the sheath into a more peripheral position. (2) Gone down the ureter? Chase it with the flexi or semirigid ureteroscope. (3) In perinephric tissue? If small (<5 mm) leave alone. (4) In a parallel lie calyx? Consider a new puncture.

Special situations

Stone and PUJ obstruction

Access via an upper pole superolateral tract provides optimum views of the PUJ. The stone is removed first and after this an endopyelotomy is performed. An endopyelotomy stent is kept in for 4 to 6 weeks.

Infundibular narrowing / stenosis

Same approach as per calyceal diverticulum (Chapter 9), i.e. puncture directly onto the stone bearing calyx. Safety wires are coiled into the calyx. The stone is cleared, then the narrowed infundibulum is dilated using either fascial or balloon dilators or forceps, once the wire has passed across the narrowing into the pelvis and down the ureter. A large nephrostomy tube is directed past the infundibulum into the pelvis or a JJ ureteric stent can be left across the infundibular narrowing.

Staghorn calculi

The different method for treating staghorn calculi are considered in Box 8.10. Figure 8.15 illustrates the difficulties in obtaining complete stone clearance with a staghorn calculi.

Sometimes numerous tracts may be required for maximal stone clearance. A combination of flexible and rigid nephroscopy with numerous retrieval devices is often required to optimise stone clearance in complex cases. Some very complex calculi are beyond endoscopic control and are better treated by anatrophic nephrolithotomy.

> **DO!** A renogram for staghorn/large calculi is recommended. If individual renal function is poor (<20%) nephrectomy should be considered

Parallel lie

A parallel lie refers to a stone within an immediately adjacent but inaccessible calyx. This situation can arise if there are a number of adjacent stone bearing calyces or if the wrong, immediately adjacent, calyx (i.e. the non-stone bearing calyx has been punctured). It is best to recognise the potential of parallel lie, and avoid it, before commencing the operation. For example if there are a number of stones in adjacent lower pole calyces, then consider whether an upper pole entry will allow navigation and stone removal from all the calyces. In the situation where there is the potenital for inaccurate targeting and inadvertent entry into the non stone bearing parallel calyx, after needle puncture and wire entry use fluoroscopic angulation and the principles of parallax (refer to Figure 5.15 and page 107 to confirm that the needle/wire are indeed in the target calyx, before track dilatation. However, once parallel lie has occurred, then a Y-track creation as demonstrated in Figure 8.16 can help retrieve the situation. It represents an elegant solution to an infrequent, but frustrating event, but it should be emphasised that this situation is best avoided in the first place.

Box 8.10 Options for staghorn calculus treatment

- PCNL monotherapy
- Combination therapy with ESWL, ESWL given after PCNL debulks the stone
- Sandwich therapy – initial PCNL followed by ESWL then a second PCNL
- PCNL two-staged procedures – with second one done during the same hospital stay or during another admission a few weeks later

---

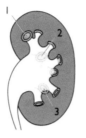

Complete Staghorn
Stone clearance may be
impossible with a single
puncture

1 Route 1 or 2 may be
   prefered – with Route 3
   PUJ/ureteric clearance
   may be difficult.
2 With either routes some
   interpolar calyces may be
   difficult.

Figure 8.15 Principles of calyceal targeting for PCNL of a complete staghorn calculus. Reproduced from Figure 2, Sandhu C, Anson KM, Patel U. Urinary tract stones – part II: current status of treatment. Clin Radiol 2003; 58: 422–33, with permission.

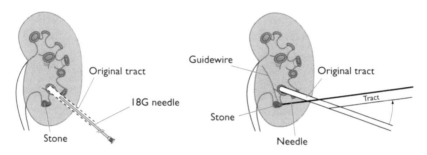

Figure 8.16 These two line drawings illustrate the creation of a Y-track for removal of a stone lying in a parallel calyx. In the first image (left) the stone is inaccessible via the existing tract. In the second image (right) the sheath has been partly withdrawn and angled towards the target parallel calyx. A needle is inserted through the re-directed sheath and used to puncture the target calyx, a wire advanced and a new tract dilated to reach the calculus. The end-result is two tracts formed but from a single skin puncture.

MINI PCNL

PCNL performed using smaller tracts (16–24F sheath) and instruments is known as mini PCNL. Proponents of this technique advocate a reduction in morbidity, although there is no evidence that a smaller tract has fewer complications. A randomised study comparing mini and standard PCNL found a significant reduction in narcotic use and hospital stay only (Feng et al., 2001). Mini PCNL requires smaller instruments that are not widely available and takes longer, especially for large stones. It is suitable for children and for small, uncomplicated stones in adults.

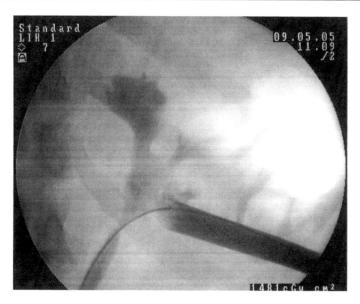

Figure 8.17 Antegrade pyelogram at end of procedure confirming stone clearance with no extravasation.

POST-EXTRACTION DRAINAGE

Following stone fragmentation and extraction, drainage of the renal unit must be secured. The commonest way is to replace the sheath with a nephrostomy tube.

Nephrostomy tubes

The type and size of the post-operative nephrostomy tube will depend upon a number of factors – the complexity of the procedure, the presence or suspicion of significant bleeding, the state of the kidney, the need for a second-look nephroscopy, the number of access tracts present and patient factors (such as obesity).

The various nephrostomy tubes available are divided according to the manner in which they are retained within the collecting system (Table 8.3 and Figure 8.18). The most widely used are the pigtail catheters, which vary in size from 5F to 22F. The Cope loop is a pigtail catheter that has a nylon string fixed between the catheter tip and the most proximal side-hole in the coil of the pigtail. Once in place, the string is pulled tight. The resulting tension leads to a tighter coil and locks the catheter from the outside.

Table 8.3 Nephrostomy tubes

Type	Retention feature	Material	Advantages	Disadvantages	Ideal use
Re-entry tube	17 cm long distal ureteric	Polyvinyl-chloride	Keeps PUJ open	Distal portion can sometimes be at VUJ	Damage or tear to PUJ
Pigtail	Distal extension coiling	Polyurethane Percuflex	Easy to insert Smaller size	Cannot do repeat nephroscopy	Simple PCNL
Kaye tamponade	36F 15 cm mechanism long balloon	Polyethylene Silitek Ultrathane Wiruthane	Allows less painful drainage and bleeding control	No tip retention through same feature tract?	Bleeding from tract
Cope loop	Extra nylon lock maintains tension of coil	Polyurethane	Secure	Need space in pelvis Pulled out whilst locked causes trauma!	Simple PCNL
U loop	Into one calyx, out of another	Silicone rubber Percuflex Silitek Ultrathane Wiruthane	Good for small renal pelvis Less encrustation Good for infundibular stenosis	Nylon can damage mucosa	Multiple tracts
Councill	Balloon	Latex	Stops catheter displacement Non-deformable loop can be exchanged over wire	Balloon can obstruct a calyx	Complicated PCNL
Malecot	Mushroom tip	Polyethylene Percuflex	Does not obstruct calyx	Retention not so secure	Uncomplicated PCNL

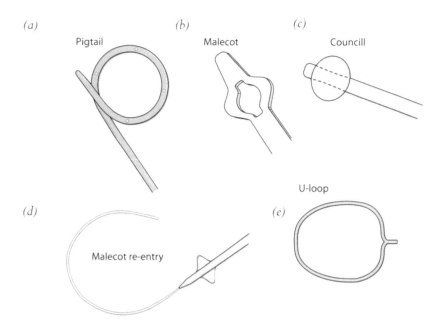

Figure 8.18 Nephrostomy drainage tubes.

Larger bore tubes only have drainage holes towards the tip and lack peripheral side-holes to avoid urinary extravasation into perinephric tissues. Councill catheters are large balloon retention catheters, and have the advantage that they can be exchanged over a guidewire. They are usually used for the complicated/bleeding cases. However, the balloon can sometimes obstruct a calyx. Malecot catheters are unlikely to obstruct as the tip is mushroom shaped instead of a balloon (Figure 8.18). The drawback is that it has a much weaker self-retaining mechanism.

When there is a large amount of bleeding from the tract, balloon tamponade catheters (Kaye tamponade catheter) allow drainage and tamponade at the same time. Re-entry tubes should be used if there is concern about keeping the PUJ open, especially if it is oedematous. They have a small ureteric extension that goes down the ureter. An endopyelotomy stent is a continuous tube that tapers to a distal segment (8F) that sits in the ureter.

The size of the nephrostomy tube depends on the viscosity of the fluid that is expected to drain and whether there may be bleeding from the tract, as a larger diameter tube will tamponade the tract. In the uncomplicated case, large sizes are unnecessary, as they will lead to more post-operative pain. Studies have shown no difference in complication rates between small (10F) and large (22F) pigtail catheters after uncomplicated PCNL (Maheshwari et al., 2000).

Tubeless PCNL

In uncomplicated cases drainage has been proposed by a ureteric catheter alone with no covering nephrostomy tube – the so-called 'tubeless PCNL' (Box 8.11).

Box 8.11 Indications for tubeless PCNL

- Smaller stone burden ($<$3 cm)
- Single puncture
- No distal obstruction
- No significant bleeding
- No collecting system perforation
- No requirement for second PCNL

(Limb & Bellman, 2002)

True tubeless PCNL

Post-procedure drainage may be avoided after a non-complicated procedure where one is confident of no obstructing residual fragments and haemorrhage has been minimal. The sheath is removed with the guidewire in place. Deep pressure is maintained with a swab on the entry site for at least 5 minutes. If the area remains dry, the guidewire can be removed and skin sutured. If there is a heavy trickle of blood, a nephrostomy tube may be inserted via the guidewire to tamponade the bleeding. The position of the tube within the collecting system must be confirmed on screening. We do not practise this and always ensure a nephrostomy tube is sited if no ureteric catheter is placed. These are subsequently removed in the early post-operative period.

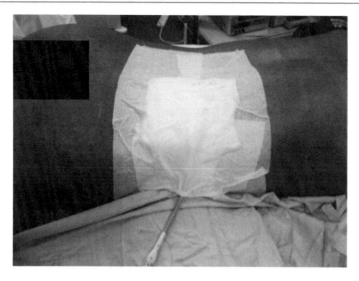

Figure 8.19 Gauze pads are folded and placed around the drainage tube in a picture frame fashion. An adhesive dressing like Mefix is placed over this.

Post-procedure care

Tubes should be sutured to the skin with a neat and firm dressing applied (Figure 8.19). Administration of local anaesthesia alongside the tube helps reduce post-operative discomfort. Box 8.12 outlines a post-operative care plan and Figure 8.20 considers the management of the post-operative nephrostomy tube.

SECOND-LOOK PROCEDURES

Second-look procedures are rarely performed, but are useful if the first procedure was complicated by bleeding, sepsis, retained calculi or anaesthetic problems and it is considered at the time that a second-look would be beneficial. A large calibre nephrostomy tube is left in the tract and a second-look procedure performed 3–5 days later by passing an Amplatz sheath over the nephrostomy tube. Often surprisingly good views are found at the second procedure and an excellent surgical outcome can result.

Box 8.12 PCNL: post-operative care plan

(1) Send stone for composition analysis and culture

(2) Hourly BP/pulse/temperature for first 6 hours – be alert for sepsis/haemorrhage

(3) Check operative site after 1–2 hours to exclude any swelling

(4) Accurate fluid balance, especially in the presence of heavy blood loss

(5) For first 24 hours maintain a good input of I.V. fluids

(6) Antibiotics – if positive culture, continue antibiotics for 5 days post-operatively. A further course of oral antibiotics for 1 to 2 weeks is warranted if difficult operation. Patients with struvite stones should receive a 6–12-week post-operative course

(7) Analgesia – opiates and anti-emetics for first 24 hours, ideally through patient controlled analgesia (PCA). Simple oral analgesia suffices afterwards. Supra-12th rib punctures are painful and inter-costal nerve blocks can be helpful in the immediate post-operative period

(8) Chest physiotherapy for supra-12th rib punctures

(9) Encourage oral fluids within first 24 hours

(10) Encourage mobilisation

(11) Remove catheters – The ureteric catheter is removed at the end of the procedure. Remove urethral catheter as soon as possible post-operatively. Keep in if required for urine output monitoring or in elderly with large obstructing prostate

---

RETAINED FRAGMENTS AND WHAT TO DO

If it is known or suspected that clinically-relevant stone fragments have been retained, then consider leaving a ureteric stent after the end of the PCNL. After the patient has recovered from the PCNL, ESWL may be tried first, preferably as an outpatient procedure. If this fails then ureterorenoscopy can be undertaken. Large fragments may require a repeat PCNL.

COMPLICATIONS

This is covered in more detail in Chapter 11, but briefly summarised in Box 8.13.

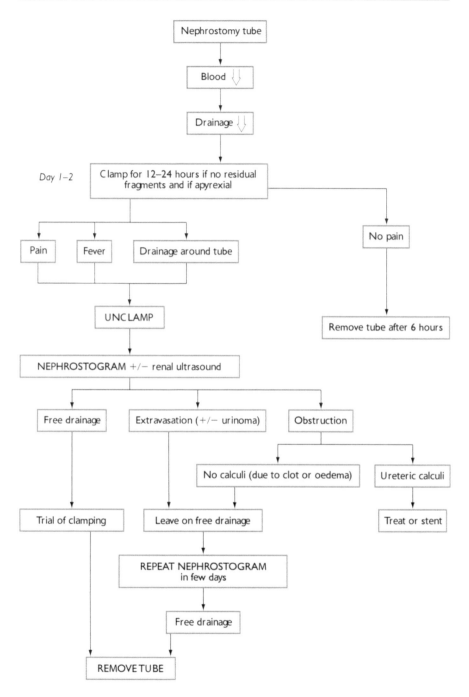

Figure 8.20 Algorithm for the post-operative management of the nephrostomy tube.

Box 8.13 PCNL complications (see Chapter 11)

(1) Major complications (2–7%)—Result in prolonged hospitalisation or require readmission to hospital for treatment. May require additional intervention and have permanent adverse sequelae. *Septic shock requiring critical care support 0.5–3%, severe acute haemorrhage <1%*

(2) Minor complications (10–25%)—Can be managed conservatively with no additional intervention and result in no permanent sequelae. *Chest complications 11%, bleeding requiring transfusion up to 2%, infundibular stenosis 2%, colonic injury 0.5%*

REFERENCES

Albala DM, Assimos DG, Clayman RV, et al. Lower pole I: a prospective randomized trial of extracorporeal shock wave lithotripsy and percutaneous nephrostolithotomy for lower pole nephrolithiasis – initial results. J Urol 2001; 166: 2072–80

Bird VG, Fallon B, Winfield HN. Practice patterns in the treatment of large renal stones. J Endourol 2003; 17: 355–63

Davidoff R, Bellman GC. Influence of technique of percutaneous tract creation on incidence of renal hemorrhage. J Urol 1997; 157: 1229–31

Feng MI, Tamaddon K, Mikhail A, et al. Prospective randomized study of various techniques of percutaneous nephrolithotomy. Urology 2001; 58: 345–50

Fernstrom I, Johansson B. Percutaneous pyelolithotomy. A new extraction technique. Scand J Urol Nephrol 1976; 10: 257–9

Kim SC, Kuo RL, Lingeman JE. Percutaneous nephrolithotomy: an update. Curr Opin Urol 2003; 13: 235–41

Kuo RL, Lingeman JE, Leveillee RJ, et al. (Lower Pole Study Group). A randomized clinical trial of ureteroscopy and percutaneous nephrolithotomy for lower pole stones between 11 and 25 mm. J Endourol 2003; 17: A31

Limb J, Bellman GC. Tubeless percutaneous renal surgery: review of first 112 patients. Urology 2002; 59: 527–31

Maheshwari PN, Andankar MG, Bansal M. Nephrostomy tube after percutaneous nephrolithotomy: large-bore or pigtail catheter? J Endourol 2000; 14: 735–7

Sandhu C, Anson KM, Patel U. Urinary tract stones – part II: current status of treatment. Clin Radiol 2003; 58: 422–33

SUGGESTED FURTHER READING

European Association of Urology. Guidelines on Urolithliasis (2001). http://www.uroweb.org/files/uploaded_files/urolithiasis.pdf

Rassweiler JJ, Renner C, Ersenberger F. The management of complex renal stones. BJU Int 2000; 86: 919–28

9. Difficult PCNLs

The previous chapter described PCNL carried out in a kidney that has ascended and rotated normally, but a characteristic of the kidney is its variable anatomy. This can make renal access and PCNL more difficult and less safe, unless the particular maldevelopment or malposition is well understood and the technique adjusted as necessary. This chapter explores the more commonly encountered variants, including the transplant kidney.

HORSESHOE KIDNEY

One in 400 of the general population has a horseshoe kidney. The condition is more common in men. The abnormal anatomy results in impaired drainage with a higher rate of calculi formation (20–50%) compared to normal kidneys. Lower pole stones are more common (Raj et al., 2003).

Anatomy

For the purposes of stone treatment some basic anatomical details should be remembered. Fusion of the lower poles during development results in a kidney that is malrotated and lies inferiorly. The anomalous rotation means that the renal pelvis is anteriorly displaced while the calyces point dorsomedially or dorsolaterally. The lower pole calyces are most medial and caudal in orientation. The blood vessels enter the kidney from the ventromedial aspect. The insertion of the ureter is high, and as a result the pelvis is longer and the PUJ is superolaterally placed. Thus many of the calyces drain poorly and some are difficult to access safely by the percutaneous route. Furthermore, intrarenal navigation is poor because of the long pelvis and its relative immobility.

Treatment

ESWL or PCNL is the treatment of choice depending on the size and location of the stone. Stones <2 cm (apart from those in an anterior mid-calyx) are treated with ESWL, but compared to ESWL in normal kidneys, ESWL has a poorer clearance and higher re-treatment rate and many operators favour PCNL as the first option. Ureterorenoscopy is technically very difficult due to the high PUJ.

Percutaneous access

Good pre-operative anatomical planning is very helpful, and this is ideally carried out with 3D CT (Ghani et al., 2005) (Figure 9.1). Upper pole access is closer to the skin surface and is the preferred route to gain access to the upper pole, lower pole and pelvis. It also minimises the torque on the kidney and thus subsequent blood loss. As the blood supply usually enters medially, the risk of bleeding is not greater than a normal kidney, as long as the puncture is posterolateral (Janetschek & Kunzel, 1988). Due to inferior displacement of the kidney, upper pole access is usually an infra-12th rib puncture (Figure 9.2). Sometimes the PCNL tract is not long enough, and there can be difficulty with instruments proving too short to reach calyceal calculi in the lower pole. Cutting out a notch at the tip of the sheath is one way of overcoming this problem. Intrarenal navigation may also be difficult as the isthmus renders the kidney relatively immobile. Access to all calyces is usually not possible with the rigid nephroscope. A working flexible nephroscope is usually therefore necessary.

Complications of PCNL in horseshoe kidneys

Up to 13% of patients will have a major complication (Raj et al., 2003; Shokeir et al., 2004). Minor complications occur in up to 20% (Raj et al., 2003). Auxiliary procedures (second look PCNL, ESWL) are required in up to a third of patients. The stone-free rate at 3 months is 90%. Up to half will form stones again (Shokeir et al., 2004).

> DO! The horseshoe kidney is predisposed to a posterolaterally displaced or retrorenal colon. Routine prone planning CT is advised to assess colonic anatomy

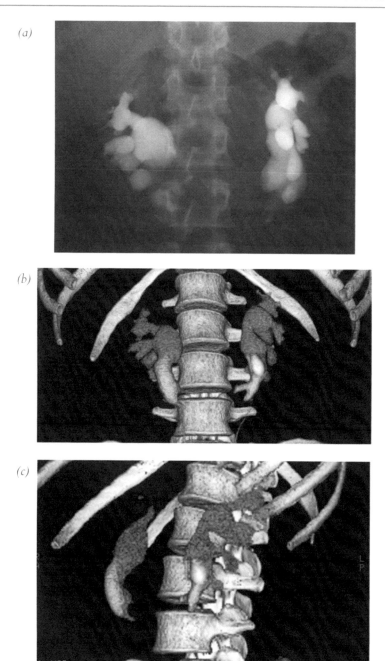

Figure 9.1 3D CT reconstruction in the planning of PCNL for horseshoe kidney.
*(a) IVU of horseshoe kidney. (b) Multislice CT urography 3D volume-rendered
reconstruction in same patient demonstrating left-sided stone. (c) Lateral view
displaying accurate 3D calyceal configuration for PCNL planning.*

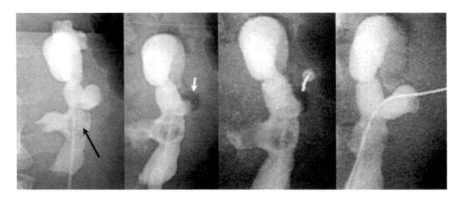

Figure 9.2 Fluoroscopic montage demonstrating a posterior calyx puncture of a horseshoe kidney in a prone patient. From left to right, the first image after retrograde injection of iodinated contrast shows the stone in the pelvis (black arrow), the next image taken after retrograde injection of air shows a posterior air-filled target calyx (white arrow), in the third image a needle is being inserted into this target calyx and the last image has been taken after complete stone removal.

PELVIC KIDNEY

Pelvic kidneys are the result of abnormality of ascend. The kidney may just be simply lower than normal, either low in the abdomen or in the pelvis, but with otherwise normal rotation. In this case the kidney is little different from a normal kidney and is treated as such. However, a pelvic kidney may also maldevelop in other ways, such that it is malrotated and/or also displaced away from the normal path of the urinary tract. At its most extreme the pelvic kidney may lie horizontally in front of the sacrum. Naturally good knowledge of the anatomical disposition is vital.

Anatomy

Congenital pelvic kidneys are more likely on the left side than the right. Unlike transplanted kidneys, which lie close to the skin surface, ectopic pelvic kidneys lie deep in the pelvis with overlying iliac vessels and intestinal loops. The orientation of an ectopic pelvic kidney is highly variable. Commonly the renal pelvis is located more medially, and some of the calyces face slightly anteriorly and could be accessed by an anterior approach or by the usually posterior route. But equally, for example with a horizontal kidney, all the calyces may be inaccessible by any route. Pre-operative anatomical planning has its obvious virtues, and CT is very useful (Figure 9.3).

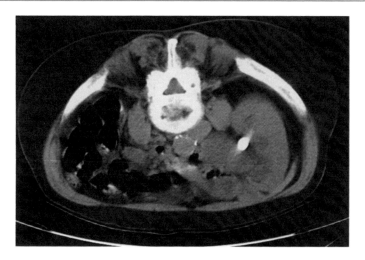

Figure 9.3 *This prone non-contrast CT demonstrates a pelvic kidney containing a stone. The pelvic bones and the bowel loops should be avoided during access.*

Treatment

Due to malrotation, ectopic kidneys are prone to recurrent stone formation, and therefore open surgery should be avoided if possible. PCNL is the recommended treatment for stones > 2 cm. Stones < 2 cm should be given ESWL in the prone position first. If ESWL fails, ureteroscopy and laser lithotripsy should be tried, although this may be technically challenging. Laparoscopic pyelolithotomy for the ectopic kidney has a high open conversion rate.

Percutaneous access

Overlying loops of bowel, and large vessels and nerves are the hurdles to safe percutaneous access. All these hazards are best appreciated on CT. Percutaneous access methods are listed in Box 9.1. The choice is best decided after careful consideration of the anatomy of the pelvic kidney.

The best-case scenario is that the CT shows a safe route without any intervening bowel loops or major vessels, in which case PCNL is carried out as normal and the chosen calyx punctured under US or fluoroscopic guidance. If, however, the safe path of entry is narrow then a two-stage procedure is carried out. First a simple nephrostomy is carried out under CT guidance to secure a safe route, and dilatation is carried out later as for the PCNL. If

---

Box 9.1 Pelvic kidney: percutaneous access methods

(1) Anterior percutaneous approach (under laparoscopic and fluoro-scopic guidance)
(2) Anterior percutaneous approach (under US guidance)
(3) Anterior percutaneous approach (under CT guidance)
(4) Posterior percutaneous approach through the greater sciatic fora-men (under fluoroscopic guidance – not for the faint hearted!) (Watterson et al., 2001)

---

there are numerous bowel loops in the way then consider the use of laparoscopy to reflect these out of the needle path. Thus each case has to be approached on its merits.

THE TRANSPLANT KIDNEY

Stones in transplanted kidneys are rare (incidence 0.1–0.2%). Predisposing risk factors include hyperparathyroidism, non-absorbable sutures, retained stents and undiscovered urolithiasis in the donor kidney (Francesca et al., 2002). The anatomy of the reconstructed ureter makes drainage of ureteric calculi difficult and, furthermore, the typical pain from renal colic does not occur due to denervation after surgery. The kidney may silently obstruct and fail, or urinary tract infection or haematuria may be the only sign of urolithiasis. Therefore a more active treatment policy is necessary for transplant kidneys. It is important to ensure stone clearance and transplanted kidneys require regular surveillance to identify recurrent calculi. Access is easier in the transplanted kidney where the renal surface is close to the anterior abdominal wall.

Anatomy

Most transplants are located in an extraperitoneal pocket in the iliac fossa. Usually the left kidney is transplanted into the right iliac fossa and vice versa. Thus the collecting system is more anterior than the renal vessels, making anterior calyceal entry safer. However, this is not invariable and in a given transplant kidney it is useful to know whether the kidney has been turned or not. The peritoneum and the bowel loops will cover most of the kidney. The ureter will have been re-implanted and ureteroscopic access may be impossible. Lastly, there is often substantial fibrosis encasing the transplant (Figure 9.4).

Treatment

Both ESWL and PCNL are options, but in either case it is important to ensure stone clearance and to guard against ureteral obstruction. A ureteric stent may be a sensible option if ESWL is used. Ureterorenoscopy is also possible if ureteral access is feasible but, because of the position and lack of mobility of the kidney, navigation may be difficult.

Percutaneous access

Important points on percutaneous access of the transplant kidney are provided in Box 9.2.

Box 9.2 Percutaneous access in the transplanted kidney

- Patient is placed in the supine position
- The side the kidney is on (usually left) is raised slightly obliquely, with a bolster placed under the hip
- The safest calyx for puncture is the most lateral and superior, as this will be away from the vessels and overlying peritoneum
- Puncture and dilatation is difficult (sometimes very difficult) due to fibrosis forming around the kidney. Navigation is also difficult because of the reduced mobility
- Mini PCNL may reduce concerns over delayed closure in immuno-suppressed patients

---

STONES IN CALYCEAL DIVERTICULUM

A calyceal diverticulum is a smooth walled cystic dilatation of the collecting system that is lined by transitional epithelium and connected to the collecting system by a narrow infundibulum. Unlike diverticula secondary to inflammatory processes such as tuberculosis, true calyceal diverticula are congenital abnormalities and are an incidental finding in up to 0.5% of the

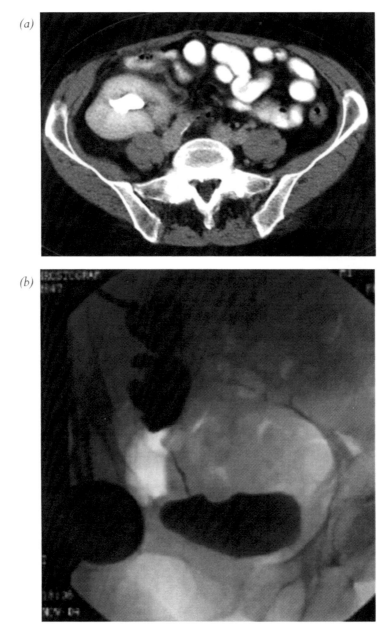

Figure 9.4 (a) Contrast CT and (b) post-PCNL nephrostogram of a transplant kidney. The particular concerns with a transplant kidney are that access should be extraperitoneal and the most lateral upper pole calyx is best. However, intrarenal navigation may be difficult as the transplant is relatively immobile. As far as possible, complete stone clearance should be the aim as retained fragments may obstruct the transplant silently.

population. As the neck of the connecting infundibulum is narrow, up to half are associated with calculi. The calculus may be entirely asymptomatic or associated with loin pain and/or recurrent urinary tract infection.

Anatomy

Most diverticulae are a branch of one of the calyces, although rarely it may branch off from the pelvis or infundibulum (pyelocalyceal diverticulum). The average size of a diverticulum varies from 0.5 to 2 cm. The majority of diverticulae are located in the upper pole and posterior facing; they may lie entirely anterior or close to major vascular divisions. Prior CT will demonstrate the relationship of the diverticulum and helps to plan the access. A further morphological, rather than strictly anatomical, consideration regarding treatment is how tightly the stone is wedged in the diverticulum. A stone that completely fills the diverticulum is much more difficult to access.

Presentation

Most diverticulae are asymptomatic. Symptoms include pain (with or without stone formation), haematuria and recurrent urinary tract infection. Abscess formation, sepsis and rupture of the parenchyma are possible sequelae of an obstructed diverticulum.

Treatment

Fewer than 50% will require operative treatment. For asymptomatic and uncomplicated diverticulae, observation is all that is required. If operative management is indicated (Box 9.3), a contrast CT scan of the abdomen can be useful to assess the size and direction of the diverticulum, size of the stone

---

Box 9.3 Indications for operative management of calyceal diverticulum

- Chronic pain
- Recurrent UTI
- Gross haematuria
- Progressive renal damage
- Increased calculus growth

(if present), the width of the neck and the thickness of the surrounding renal parenchyma. These factors guide treatment choices (Table 9.1).

Percutaneous management

This is the optimum method for attaining stone-free and symptom-free results, with results exceeding 80% (Shalhav et al., 1998). The aim of treat-

Table 9.1 Stone in calyceal diverticulum: treatment options

Treatment option	Indications	Advantages	Disadvantages
ESWL	• Small stone burden (<1 cm) • Wide-necked diverticula	• Less morbidity	• Poor stone clearance rate • Does not obliterate abnormal anatomy therefore high stone recurrence rate
Ureteroscopy	• <1.5 cm stone burden • Anterior facing diverticula • Middle/upper pole location	• Less morbidity • Preferable in patients with significant co-morbidities • Able to dilate neck of diverticulum (technically difficult)	• Difficult to identify diverticular ostium • Difficult to obliterate cavity • Considerably poorer stone-free and symptom-free rates compared to PCNL
Percutaneous	• Large stone burden (>1.5 cm) • Lower pole location • Posterior diverticulum	• Obliteration of cavity • High stone-free and symptom-free rates	• Greater morbidity
Laparoscopic	• Thin renal parenchyma overlying the diverticulum • Anterior facing diverticula	• Obliteration of cavity • Option to nephrectomy possible in presence of suspicious macropathology	• Greater morbidity • Relatively new technique which may be technically difficult

ment is to obtain complete stone clearance with ablation of the cavity or dilatation of its connection with the collecting system, in order to prevent future stone recurrence.

Percutaneous access

Direct approach

This involves a puncture directly onto the stone-bearing calyceal diverticulum. Ideally, a curved-tipped hydrophilic wire is manipulated through the ostium of the diverticulum into the renal pelvis (Figure 9.5).

Distension (via the ureteric catheter) during wire manipulation helps, however this manoeuvre may fail and the guidewire has to be coiled into several loops within the diverticulum to maintain access. Great skill is needed to keep the coils in place and not lose access to the collecting system during tract dilatation (Figure 9.6).

Dilatation is best carried out with the metal telescopic dilators as they have a zero tip and, with care, can be carefully placed to just within the diverticulum. If the renal parenchyma is thin, it may be difficult to stabilise the guidewire within the cavity. A large stone can make it difficult to coil the wire or traverse the infundibulum.

> **DO!** Use a curved tip hydrophilic wire and saline distension to manipulate the wire through the tight ostium

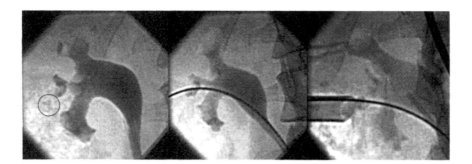

Figure 9.5 Intra-operative images of PCNL of a stone-bearing calyceal diverticulum. From left to right, the first image shows a stone in a tight diverticulum (circle), in the next image after direct puncture onto the stone a hydrophilic wire has been manipulated across the neck of the diverticulum and in the last image after dilatation using metal (zero-tip) dilators a 30F working sheath has been advanced up to the diverticulum.

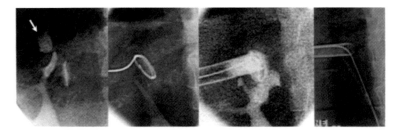

Figure 9.6 From left to right, the first image shows an upper pole calyx (arrowed) with a stone (not seen on this image), the next shows that a wire is coiled in the diverticulum, the third shows that after metal dilatation a sheath has been carefully advanced up to the diverticulum without losing wire access. In the last image after stone removal a wire has been advanced through the neck of the diverticulum under direct endoscopic vision prior to dilatation of the neck.

If the guidewire cannot be passed through the ostium into the pelvis or coiled within the diverticulum, a neoinfundibulutomy can be created to gain access to the renal pelvis (Auge et al., 2002) (Figure 9.7). A percutaneous access needle is passed from the inner diverticulum wall through the medullary portion of the parenchyma into the renal pelvis. A guidewire is passed through this needle, and secured down the ureter. The tract is dilated to 30F with a balloon catheter. This technique carries the risk of haemorrhage from the interlobar arteries. However, in the series reported by Auge and colleagues no major complications were noted.

Indirect approach
Access is obtained through a separate calyx, and a flexible nephroscope is used to get a guidewire past the ostium of the diverticulum. The neck is dilated or incised with the holmium laser.

Dilating the neck of the diverticulum

After removal of the stone, forceps (Figure 9.8) or dilators (balloon or fascial up to 14F) may be used to open up the ostium and access the main collecting system.

> DO! Retrograde injection of methylene blue through the ureteric catheter can help locate a hard to find ostium

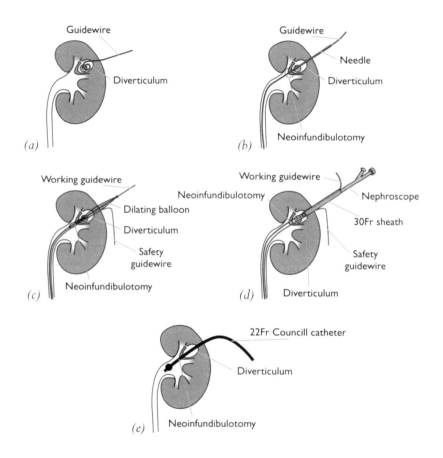

Figure 9.7 Neoinfundibulutomy: calyceal diverticulum containing stone with stenotic infundibulum into upper pole calyx. (a) Guidewire has been introduced into diverticulum percutaneously without success in traversing infundibulum. (b) Needle has been re-introduced and advanced through diverticulum and renal parenchyma directly into renal pelvis, creating neoinfundibulutomy. Guidewire is then passed into ureter through needle. (c) Two guidewires have been introduced into ureter through neoinfundibulutomy, which is subsequently dilated with standard 30F balloon dilator. (d) Nephroscopy sheath is advanced under fluoroscopic guidance over balloon into renal pelvis. Sheath and nephroscope are then withdrawn from pelvis into calyceal diverticulum for stone fragmentation and diverticular fulguration. (e) At end of procedure 22F Councill catheter is placed over working wire with tip of catheter situated in renal pelvis. Reproduced from Auge BK, et al. Neoinfundibulotomy for the management of symptomatic caliceal diverticula. J Urol 2002; 167: 1616–20, with permission.

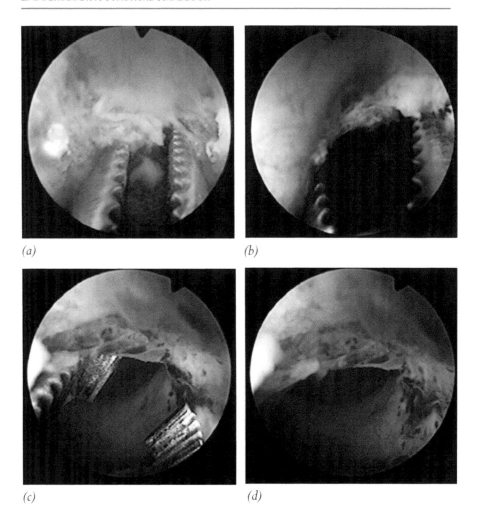

Figure 9.8 (a) to (d) Endoscopic images taken during PCNL depicting forceps dilatation of the ostium of a calyceal diverticulum.

DO! If electrocautery is used, a safety wire should be inserted with an open-ended catheter to prevent transmission down the ureter

Ablation of cavity

Small diverticula (<2.5 cm) do not require fulguration since the trauma of dilatation is felt to be enough to bring about obliteration of the cavity. Superficial fulguration to the lining of the diverticular cavity and neck may be achieved using the holmium laser or electrocautery with a Bugbee wire or rollerball on a transurethral resectoscope. Ablation of a wide-neck infundibulum is often difficult and is at risk of prolonged post-operative urinary leak.

Post-extraction drainage

If the neck has been dilated, a nephrostomy tube should be placed through the diverticulum into the renal pelvis and be kept in place for 24–48 hours. If the neck has not been opened, a nephrostomy tube is placed into the diverticulum with a double J stent in the ureter. If a neoinfundibulutomy tract has been created, the tube should remain in for a week to allow epithelialisation.

Flexible ureterorenoscopy (flexi URS)

The entrance to the diverticulum may be incised using the holmium laser. The neck may be also be dilated using a zero-tip balloon catheter, although it can be difficult to maintain adequate deflection with the scope in order to place a balloon dilator through the orifice. If access is feasible, good stone-free rates of 60% are achievable with flexible URS (Batter & Dretler, 1997). However, the difficulty with flexi URS lies with identifying and accessing the ostium of the diverticulum, as well as achieving obliteration of the cavity. A combined flexi URS and percutaneous approach may be used to place a guidewire through the ostium using flexi URS, which is brought out retrogradely for percutaneous access.

Laparoscopy

Laparoscopic unroofing and ablation is ideal for large diverticula with surrounding thin renal parenchyma. A retroperitoneal approach is suitable for posterior facing diverticula, whilst transperitoneal is suitable for anterior. The diverticulum may be identified using fluoroscopy, retrograde injection of methylene blue or laparoscopic ultrasound. The diverticulum can be obliterated by suturing or argon beam coagulation. This is a relatively new technique and experience is limited (Miller et al., 2002).

FURTHER DIFFICULT PCNLs

Kyphoscoliosis

As a result of severe thoraco-lumbar spinal deformity the kidney may be displaced and/or malrotated. In extreme cases the kidney may lie in the pelvis. The anatomical limitations are similar to those discussed with pelvic and horseshoe kidneys. Our policy is to ensure that we have maximal anatomical information prior to the PCNL. Essentially this means a CT carried out in the prone position (Figure 9.9).

Stone treatment is worthwhile in these patients as complications can occur silently because of decreased sensation. PCNL is the ideal option but, as well as the anatomical limitations discussed above, navigation is difficult because of the restricted space and there is an increased risk of sepsis.

Pregnancy

Successful PCNL has been reported during pregnancy, but with the advent of flexible ureterorenoscopy the need for this is even less now.

Large spleen

CT- or ultrasound-guided puncture will be required if splenomegaly is present. Once access into the pelvicalyceal system is safely secured, dilatation and stone treatment can continue as for a normal kidney (Beale et al., 1997).

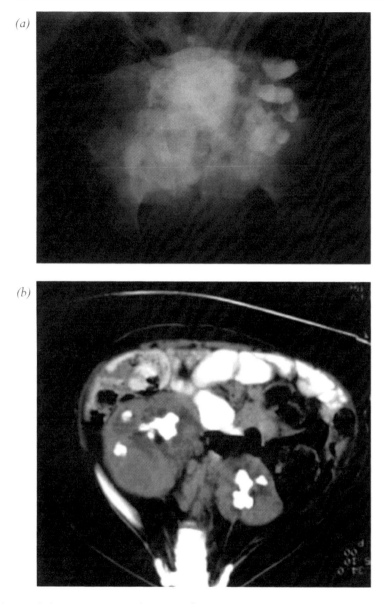

(a)

(b)

Figure 9.9 An IVU (a) and CT (b) of a patient with spina bifida and severe kyphoscoliosis.

REFERENCES

Auge BK, Munver R, Kourambas J, et al. Neoinfundibulotomy for the management of symptomatic caliceal diverticula. J Urol 2002; 167: 1616–20

Batter SJ, Dretler SP. Ureterorenoscopic approach to the symptomatic caliceal diverticulum. J Urol 1997; 158: 709–13

Beale TJ, Anson K, Watson M, Kellett MJ, Allen C. Massive splenomegaly complicating left percutaneous renal surgery. Br J Urol 1997; 80: 829–30

Francesca F, Felipetto R, Mosca F, et al. Percutaneous nephrolithotomy of transplanted kidney. J Endourol 2002; 16: 225–7

Ghani KR, Rintoul M, Patel U, Anson K. Three-dimensional planning of percutaneous renal stone surgery in a horseshoe kidney using 16-slice CT and volume-rendered movies. J Endourol 2005; 19: 461–3

Janetschek G, Kunzel KH. Percutaneous nephrolithotomy in horseshoe kidneys. Applied anatomy and clinical experience. Br J Urol 1988; 62: 117–22

Miller SD, Ng CS, Streem SB, et al. Laparoscopic management of caliceal diverticular calculi. J Urol 2002; 167: 1248–52

Raj GV, Auge BK, Weizer AZ, et al. Percutaneous management of calculi within horseshoe kidneys. J Urol 2003; 170: 48–51

Shalhav AL, Soble JJ, Nakada SY, et al. Long-term outcome of caliceal diverticula following percutaneous endosurgical management. J Urol 1998; 160: 1635–9

Shokeir AA, El-Nahas AR, Shoma AM, et al. Percutaneous nephrolithotomy in treatment of large stones within horseshoe kidneys. Urology 2004; 64: 426–9

Watterson JD, Cook A, Sahajpal R, et al. Percutaneous nephrolithotomy of a pelvic kidney: a posterior approach through the greater sciatic foramen. J Urol 2001; 166: 209–10

SUGGESTED FURTHER READING

Canales B, Monga M. Surgical management of the calyceal diverticulum. Curr Opin Urol 2003; 13: 255–60

Crook TJ, Keoghane SR. Renal transplant lithiasis: rare but time-consuming. BJU Int 2005; 95: 931–3

10. Upper Urinary Tract TCC

Upper urinary tract transitional cell carcinoma (TCC) is rare, accounting for 2–5% of all urothelial cancers. The overwhelming majority of upper tract primary urothelial tumours are TCC. Squamous cell carcinoma and adenocarcinoma constitute the remainder, and may be associated with chronic infection (*schistosoma haematobium*) or stones.

Improvements in flexible ureterorenoscopy (flexi URS) and ancillary instrumentation have made endoscopic management of upper tract TCC possible, with a consequent reduction in morbidity and preservation of the functioning renal unit. The techniques that have been developed for endoscopic management of lower tract TCC are now being translated to the upper tract. There is now considerable interest in the role of endoscopic management of this disease in appropriately selected patients. The picture is evolving all the time as centres across the world develop the expertise needed to diagnose and treat upper tract TCC.

PATHOPHYSIOLOGY

Upper tract TCC is a result of a genetic field defect leading to multiple recurrences in varied locations on the urothelium over time (polychronotopism). Multifocal lesions are present in up to a third of patients on presentation and these patients have a poorer prognosis as the tumours are often muscle invasive at the time of diagnosis. The tendency for polychronotopism is confined mostly to the ipsilateral renal unit. As a result, synchronous and metachronous involvement of the contralateral renal unit is rare (1% and 2–4%, respectively) (Mills et al., 2001). The relationship between upper and lower tract TCC is illustrated in Figure 10.1.

Macropathological features of upper tract TCC are similar to bladder TCC. Papillary tumours are the predominant type (Figure 10.1), followed by sessile and flat lesions. The risk factors for developing TCC are listed in Box 10.1. In most societies smoking remains the most significant risk factor for TCC.

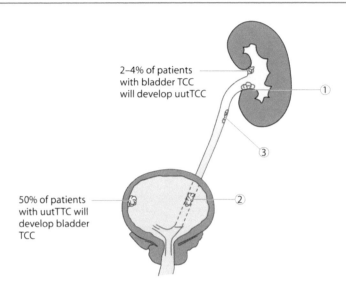

Figure 10.1 Relationship between upper tract TCC and bladder TCC. The most common site of uut TCC is in the renal pelvis (1) followed by the distal (2), then proximal ureter (3).

Box 10.1 Risk factors for developing TCC

(1) Smoking
(2) Exposure to occupational carcinogens (aromatic amines and aniline dyes)
(3) Analgesic abuse (phenacetin)
(4) Chronic administration of cyclophosphamide
(5) Balkan nephropathy

PRESENTATION

Haematuria (macro/microscopic) is the cardinal feature of upper tract TCC. Some patients may present with flank pain due to obstruction from a ureteral or pelvic tumour or from clot passage. Tumours may also be diagnosed during upper tract TCC surveillance, after positive urine cytology and a negative cystoscopy and biopsy, or after discovery of a filling defect on an IVU or loopogram.

(a)

(b)

(c)

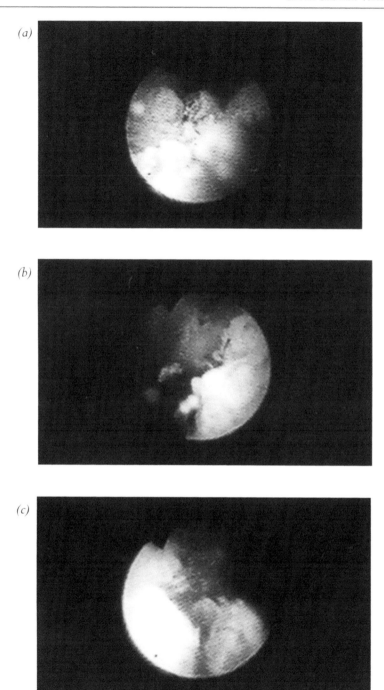

Figure 10.2 *(a) to (c) Flexible URS images of a predominantly solid TCC in the renal pelvis with some papillary elements. This was a G3pT2 lesion.*

INVESTIGATIONS

Haematuria warrants immediate investigation with cystoscopy, voided urine cytology and upper tract imaging. Plain abdominal radiography (KUB) and renal tract ultrasound are the imaging modalities of choice presently, but if investigations are negative or equivocal then an IVU is indicated. The majority of upper tract TCC will be diagnosed as filling defects on IVU (Figure 10.3). Currently the role of CT urography and MR urography is being investigated, and it is predicted that, with the necessary technical improvements, these techniques will replace the IVU for upper tract imaging. However, in all cases, diagnostic ureterorenoscopy is then indicated for biopsy confirmation and cellular staging.

Urine cytology

Voided urine cytology has poor sensitivity for low/moderate grade upper tract TCC unless the lesion is carcinoma *in situ* (CIS) or high grade. This is because of the higher rate of desquamation of these cells. The diagnostic yield can be significantly increased if selective upper tract urine cytology is performed using a ureteral catheter (aspiration or saline barbotage cytology), with sensitivities approaching 80% (Zincke et al., 1976). Brushings (Figure 10.4) can increase the sensitivity and specificity of cytological analysis to 91% and 94% respectively (Dodd et al., 1997). Employing molecular

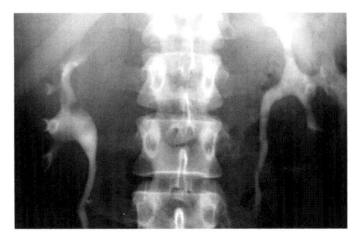

Figure 10.3 IVU of uut TCC detected as a filling defect in the infundibulum of the upper pole of the right kidney.

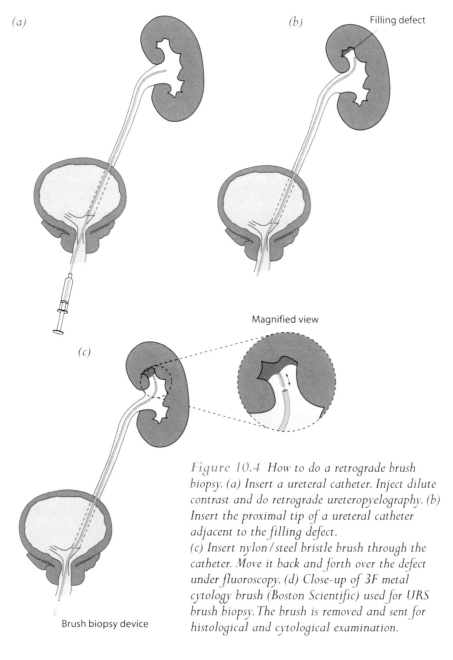

(a)

(b) Filling defect

(c)

Magnified view

Brush biopsy device

Figure 10.4 *How to do a retrograde brush biopsy. (a) Insert a ureteral catheter. Inject dilute contrast and do retrograde ureteropyelography. (b) Insert the proximal tip of a ureteral catheter adjacent to the filling defect.*
(c) Insert nylon/steel bristle brush through the catheter. Move it back and forth over the defect under fluoroscopy. (d) Close-up of 3F metal cytology brush (Boston Scientific) used for URS brush biopsy. The brush is removed and sent for histological and cytological examination.

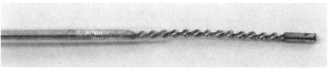

(d)

techniques such as p53 nuclear protein immunostaining may also increase diagnostic sensitivity (Keeley et al., 1997).

Imaging

Retrograde ureteropyelography can confirm the presence of a known filling defect or discover further abnormalities (Figure 10.5). Ultrasound and CT can exclude other causes of filling defects such as stones and blood clot. A CT of the abdomen/pelvis provides preoperative staging information when upper tract TCC is suspected. However, CT is unable to distinguish local stage accurately, especially between Ta and T2 lesions (Figure 10.6). Endoluminal ultrasound is capable of providing information about depth of invasion, but has not made much practical impact as it is technically difficult.

Flexible ureterorenoscopy (flexi URS)

Endoscopy is the gold standard investigation for suspected upper tract TCC, with diagnostic sensitivity approaching 100% in experienced hands. The

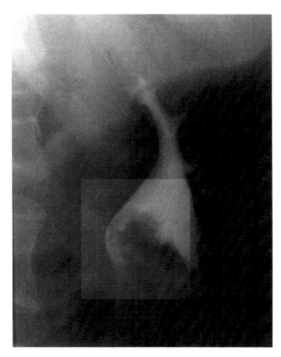

Figure 10.5 A retrograde pyelogram showing a filling defect in the renal pelvis due to a transitional cell carcinoma.

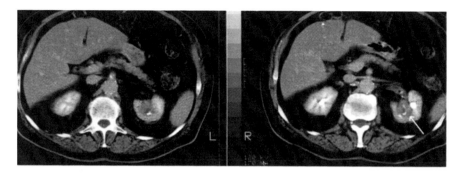

Figure 10.6 Axial CT scans demonstrating a left-sided TCC of the renal pelvis (arrow).

miniaturisation of fibreoptic endoscopes has resolved previous access difficulties. In particular, with flexi URS complete inspection of the upper urinary tract is now possible. As well as providing a visual assessment, flexi URS allows for biopsy and assessment of tumour grade and stage. The latter is less reliable, especially in the ureter where the thin wall limits extensive biopsy. It should be remembered that currently biopsy commonly understages upper tract tumours.

Grade and stage

Cytological and histological examination guides treatment and prognosis. Studies have shown excellent correlation between biopsy grade and final resected specimen grade. The correlation between tumour grade and stage (Table 10.1) is such that the grade of the biopsy is used to guide definitive treatment (Keeley et al, 1997a) i.e. high-grade tumours on biopsy are more likely to be high-stage tumours. Low-grade tumours that are not invasive on CT are likely to be superficial tumours, and it is these tumours that are most suitable for endoscopic management. The 1973 WHO classification system is the most widely used grading system, and is based on the worst grade seen (Table 10.2). The 1998 WHO/International Society of Urologic Pathology classification system is a slightly modified classification system for grading urothelial tumours. Molecular staging techniques may also be helpful in guiding treatment. Adverse prognostic molecular markers include DNA aneuploidy, E-cadherin underexpression, EGF and c-erb-B-2 oncoprotein expression (Mills et al., 2001).

Table 10.1 TNM system for staging upper tract TCC

Tumour	Nodes	Metastases
Tx Primary tumour cannot be assessed	NX Regional lymph nodes cannot be assessed	Mx Distant metastasis cannot be assessed
T0 No evidence of primary tumour	N0 No regional lymph node metastasis	M0 No distant metastasis
Ta Papillary non-invasive	N1 Metastasis in a single node ≤ 2 cm	M1 Distant metastasis
Tis CIS		
T1 Invades subepithelial connective tissue	N2 Metastasis in a single node between 2–5 cm in size or multiple nodes <5 cm in size each	
T2 Invades the muscularis		
T3 Renal pelvis: invades beyond muscularis into peripelvic fat or parenchyma	N3 Metastasis in a lymph node >5 cm in size	
T3 Ureter: invades beyond muscularis into periureteric fat		
T4 Invades adjacent organs or into perinephric fat		

Table 10.2 TCC grade classification

WHO classification 1973	WHO/International Society of Urologic Pathology 1998
Grade 1 (well differentiated)	Papillary urothelial tumours of low malignant potential (LMP)
Grade 2 (moderately differentiated)	Low-grade (LG) urothelial carcinoma
Grade 3 (poorly differentiated)	High-grade (HG) urothelial carcinoma

TIP! Grade 2 tumours should be treated as potentially invasive

MANAGEMENT

Treatment is based upon grade and stage of TCC at the time of diagnosis. Open nephroureterectomy has been the standard treatment for upper tract TCC. Radical laparoscopic and conservative endoscopic surgery are relatively new procedures that are becoming increasingly popular and it is likely that laparoscopic techniques will replace traditional open nephroureterectomy.

RADICAL SURGERY

Open nephroureterectomy

Due to the multifocal and recurrent nature of upper tract TCC, the treatment of choice is open radical nephroureterectomy with removal of bladder cuff around the ipsilateral ureteral orifice. Nephroureterectomy is the gold standard due to the higher rate of cancer-free survival and high recurrence rates evident with conservative nephron-sparing procedures.

Laparoscopic nephroureterectomy

In many centres this is now the preferred method for treating upper tract TCC. The approach may be either transperitoneal or retroperitoneal. The distal ureter with a bladder cuff can be removed laparoscopically or through an open approach. If a wholly laparoscopic approach is used, a small incision in the flank or suprapubic port site is required to remove the specimen intact.

Compared to open surgery, laparoscopic nephroureterectomy has been conclusively shown to reduce blood loss, patient morbidity and hospital stay, and to result in shorter patient recovery times. A Medline review of laparoscopic nephroureterectomy performed over a 13-year period showed it to be equal to open surgery with respect to oncological outcomes of 5-year survival, local recurrence rates and positive surgical margins. The only exception was the incidence of port site metastasis: 1.6% of patients developed port site metastasis within 12 months of laparoscopic surgery (Rassweiler et al., 2004). It is likely that with a refinement of technique with watertight en bloc dissection this figure will be comparable with open outcomes.

CONSERVATIVE NEPHRON-SPARING SURGERY

Open segmental resection

Where the aim of surgery has been renal preservation, low-grade/stage tumours of the distal ureter have been treated by open distal ureterectomy incorporated with ureteric re-implantation via a Boari flap or hitch. This open method of conservation has been more or less abandoned with the advent of sophisticated endoscopic techniques.

Endoscopic treatment

Endoscopic management of upper tract TCC was initially introduced as a method for treating patients requiring renal unit preservation in order to avoid dialysis. It has now evolved into a procedure suitable for certain patients with normal contralateral kidneys (Table 10.3). Low-grade/stage tumours that are accessible may be treated by endoscopic resection and ablation (Box 10.2). High-grade tumours and CIS are very difficult to treat endoscopically and should be treated by nephroureterectomy. Before embarking on endoscopic treatment, patients need to be informed of the implications of endoscopic management and must submit to life-long endoscopic, radiological and cytological surveillance.

The choice between retrograde or antegrade endoscopic resection is dependent upon tumour size, multiplicity and location. Ureterorenoscopy is the preferred choice because of the lower morbidity and the ability to maintain the integrity of the upper tract. A preoperative checklist prior to endoscopic resection is provided in Box 10.3.

Table 10.3 Indications for endoscopic management of upper tract TCC	
Absolute indications	*Relative indications*
• Solitary kidney	In the presence of a normal
• Renal insufficiency in contralateral kidney	contralateral kidney:
• Bilateral TCC	• Low grade (G1–2) lesions
• Co-morbidities that contraindicate	• Size (less than <2 cm)
open/laparoscopic surgery	
• Palliation	

Box 10.2 Thinking of endoscopic surgery? Factors to consider

- Tumour grade
- Location of tumour
- Size of tumour

Box 10.3 Endoscopic resection of upper tract TCC: preoperative checklist

---

(1) *Consent:* patient understands reasons for endoscopic management and agrees to life-long surveillance. Aware of complications like perforation and stricture formation, and the possibility of stent insertion. Consent for conversion to open surgery in case of uncontrollable bleeding

(2) *Imaging:* review previous IVU, retrograde studies and CT scan if available. Be aware of the anatomy of the upper tract and size, location and number of lesions

(3) *Urine:* know recent culture and voided cytology results

(4) *Fluoroscopy:* technicians notified and image intensifier available for procedure

(5) *Mark:* put an arrow in the lower flank of the correct side with indelible ink

(6) *Pathology:* liaise closely with pathologist (may need frozen section and cytopreparations)

URETERORENOSCOPIC MANAGEMENT OF UPPER TRACT TCC

Principles of ureteroscopy

The operative steps for endoscopic management of upper tract TCC are summarised in Box 10.5. If not already performed, the procedure should start with a rigid cystoscopy to exclude synchronous bladder TCC and collection of bladder urine for cytology if unavailable. A ureteric catheter is inserted and retrograde ureteropyelography should be performed to delineate the anatomy of the upper tract.

> **DO!** Dilute contrast medium to 30–50% to reveal subtle filling defects during retrograde ureteropyelography

The ureter should be inspected with minimal trauma as far as possible using a small calibre (6.9F) semirigid ureteroscope. This should be done preferably without a guidewire to avoid ureteral trauma, the so called 'no touch' technique. Ureteral trauma has undesirable outcomes that effect the diagnostic sensitivity of ureteroscopy (Box 10.4).

Box 10.4 Reasons for 'no touch' URS technique

(1) Traumatic mucosa may be mistaken for a pathological lesion
(2) Trauma also increases the false-positive rate of upper tract biopsies because of artifactual change in cell morphology from instrumentation
(3) Bleeding from trauma obscures vision and reduces the diagnostic sensitivity of ureterorenoscopy

---

> **DO!** Use low-pressure irrigation to reduce the risk of tumour migration from pyelovenous, pyelolymphatic or pyelotubular backflow

---

Box 10.5 URS for upper tract TCC: operative steps

(1) Retrograde study
(2) Semirigid URS
(3) Upper tract cytology
(4) Insert guidewire
(5) Flexi URS
(6) Navigation of entire upper tract
(7) Barbotage cytology from around lesion
(8) Biopsy lesion
(9) Resect/vaporise then fulgurate/ablate (if typical appearance of TCC)
(10) Ureteric stent inserted if needed

The entire ureter should be inspected in this manner with the semirigid ureteroscope, after which a guidewire can be inserted up to the level reached by the scope, but not beyond. The semirigid scope may then be removed with the guidewire in place. The flexi URS is then inserted over the guidewire in a monorail fashion under direct vision and screening, to inspect the rest of the ureter and the intrarenal collecting system.

Diagnosis

The entire urothelium must be inspected in a systematic manner. Diluted contrast material should be injected into the renal pelvis and a road map of the intrarenal collecting system should be drawn along with any filling defects. All calyces should be entered with the flexible endoscope, starting from the upper pole and working downwards to the lower pole. The number and location of lesions identified should be charted (see Chapter 4 on how to do a 'road map'). Visual inspection can differentiate between other causes of filling defects. Tumours may be distinguished by their appearance.

A specimen of urine for cytology can be obtained from the upper tract through the semirigid ureteroscope. Additional urine can be aspirated surrounding a lesion or near a filling defect through the working channel of the ureteroscope using 10 ml of normal saline (barbotage cytology). Tumour biopsy should be performed using either a 2.5F flat wire basket for papillary lesions (Figure 10.7) or a 3F cup biopsy forceps for flat lesions. Further urine can be aspirated after biopsy.

DON'T! Don't crush tissue with the basket by closing it tightly as this makes pathological diagnosis more difficult

---

DO! Consider performing contralateral ureteric washings and imaging if clinical suspicion of contralateral disease is high

---

Treatment

Superficial papillary lesions suggestive of TCC may be resected and ablated at the same procedure. If doubts remain as to the nature of the lesion a frozen section may be taken. Resection may be carried out using either

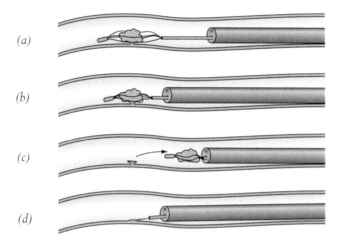

Figure 10.7 How to biopsy with a basket. (a) Basket (flat-wire) is put over the lesion under direct vision and/or fluoroscopy. (b) Basket closed over lesion/filling defect and kept closed under vision. (c) Remove basket with scope. Whole basket with specimen put in container and sent to pathology. Place large specimens in formalin and small (<1 mm) in saline. (d) Return with laser fibre or Bugbee electrode and coagulate the bed of the lesion.

electrosurgery or laser surgery. Most patents will require more than one procedure to render them tumour-free. A ureteric stent should be inserted if there has been a perforation or when resection has been extensive. When an intrarenal tumour is inaccessible, or is too large to be resected using URS, a percutaneous approach should be considered. In a minority, even after multiple procedures, endoscopic surgery will fail to remove the entire tumour.

ELECTROSURGERY

Resection with loop resectoscope

The larger size of this rigid instrument (11.5F) limits its applications in the confined spaces of the ureter (Figure 10.8a). The irrigation fluid must be changed to glycine or sorbitol. Tissue is resected using the same principles employed when working in the lower tract. Cutting energy is put to the lowest setting that produces adequate resection, otherwise perforation is the consequence. Small loops of tissue must be taken slowly. The procedure can take time and the scope may need to be withdrawn at intervals to clear tissue from the resectoscope loop. After resection the base should be lightly fulgurated.

The drawback with loop resection is the large size of the instrument, which limits access and increases the incidence of stricture formation (Figure 10.9). Pure cut without blend and no coagulation during resection will help minimise post-operative stricture formation.

DO! Avoid conducting current and inadvertently coagulating the ureter. Use a Teflon-sheathed nitinol guidewire instead of a PTFE wire

---

DON'T! Unlike bladder mucosa, ureteric mucosa strictures easily. Avoid excessive fulguration to the tumour base as this leads to scarring and stricture formation

---

(a)

(b)   (c)

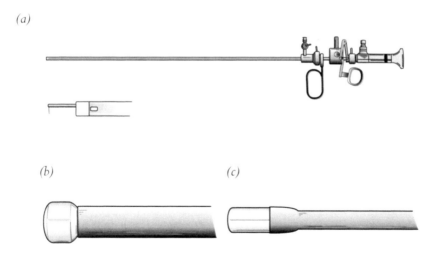

Figure 10.8 Equipment for electrosurgical ablation of urothelial lesions. (a) Uretero-resectoscope with inset showing hook electrode for loop resection. (b) Bugbee flexible coagulation electrode – 'button' type (size 5F). (c) Bugbee electrode suitable for flexi URS – 'straight' type (size 3F). (All courtesy of RichardWolf UK Ltd)

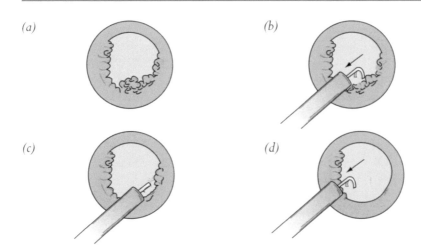

Figure 10.9 Resecting tumours that are more than 50% of the ureteral circumference increases the risk of stricture formation. These tumours should be resected by a two-stage operation, in order to allow the resected ureter to heal in the interval. (a) Tumour exceeds 50% of circumference. (b) Half of tumour resected. (c) Bugbee electrode to coagulate base of tumour. (d) Remainder of tumour resected at a later stage.

Fulguration with Bugbee electrode

With the Bugbee electrode, smaller lesions and the base of large tumours can be fulgurated. They are available in sizes ranging from 2 to 5F. The 2F or 3F probe can be used during flexi URS (Figure 10.8b,c).

LASER SURGERY

Laser energy can be delivered through miniature flexible fibres via both flexible and semirigid URS. The advantages of laser surgery compared to electrosurgery, are a lower stricture rate and the ability to use normal saline as the irrigation fluid. The most widely used lasers are neodymium: yttrium–aluminium–garnet (Nd:YAG) and holmium:YAG (see Table 10.4). Both are equally effective in destroying tumours (Figure 10.10).

Table 10.4 Laser surgery for upper tract TCC

	Nd:YAG	Ho:YAG
Fibre size	200 – 400 μm	200 or 365 μm
Energy setting	10–30 W Continuous wave pulses	Laser is activated to 0.6 to 1.2 J Frequency of pulsation 5–10 Hz
Depth of penetration	5–8 mm	0.5 mm
Technique	• Direct fibre at tumour – remain close but free beam not contact • Avoid contact with tip when activated or lip will char • Move tip over surface to 'paint' coagulation • Parallel fire to ureteral wall lowers risk of perforation in ureter	• Requires tissue contact • Lower energy over tissue whilst bleeding will give a more diffuse effect
Advantages	• Greater depth of penetration for treating bulkier tumours • Suitable for large vascular tumours • Deep coagulative effect	• Energy observed only tissue effect achieved – 'what you see is what you get' • Coagulate, ablate and remove tissue • Pinpoint accuracy • Open up lumen if occlusive neoplasm • Good haemostasis • Limited penetration so good for near vessel work • Minimal stricturing • Better for circumferential lesions
Disadvantages	• Forward scatter risk • Higher risk of stricture and perforation	• Low tissue penetration • Often need to completely clear field of tissue debris

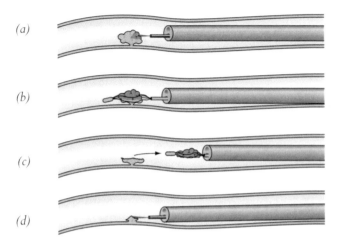

Figure 10.10 *Resecting tumour with the laser. (a) Fire laser and coagulate the top of the tumour. (b) and (c) Coagulated tissue is removed with either a basket (flat-wire) or forceps. (d) Further laser energy for base of tumour.*

COMPLICATIONS OF RETROGRADE ENDOSCOPIC SURGERY

Perforation

Perforation is a possible consequence when resecting a mucosal lesion from the ureter. The perforation rate reported in the published literature ranges from 0 to 10%. Perforation is less common in the distal ureter where the wall is relatively thick and immobile. Modern-day series show a much lower rate of perforation due to the miniaturisation of equipment and increasing popularity of the holmium laser. Most if not all perforations can be managed conservatively with stenting for 2 to 3 weeks to reduce the risk of stricture formation.

Stricture

The reported incidence of stricture formation following endoscopic management of upper tract TCC varies from 0 to 16%. Factors that affect stricture formation include the extent of resection and energy source used for resection and ablation (Box 10.6). The introduction of holmium laser tumour ablation has contributed to a reduction in the incidence of post-operative stricture. Strictures may be treated with balloon incision or dilatation and stent placement.

DO! Do not assume strictures are a complication of treatment. Always biopsy to exclude malignancy

---

Box 10.6 Stricture formation: risk factors

- Electrosurgery
- Excision of circumferential tumours
- Previous multiple URS
- Resection over ureteric orifice
- Previous BCG treatment
- Previous radiation therapy

Extraluminal spillage of tumour

Ureteroscopy and biopsy do not affect tumour recurrence. Studies have shown no difference in recurrence rates in patients undergoing radical surgery after URS and biopsy (Hendin et al., 1999). Although tumour seeding after perforation during ureteroscopy has not been reported, high irrigation pressures should be avoided during the procedure.

PERCUTANEOUS MANAGEMENT OF UPPER TRACT TCC

Percutaneous surgery for upper tract TCC permits superior visibility and resection due to larger instrumentation. Indications for percutaneous management of upper tract TCC are listed in Table 10.5. The percutaneous approach more or less guarantees access to the upper tract urothelium in situations where retrograde access is difficult. However, this is offset by greater morbidity and longer hospital stay compared with flexi URS treatment. Another disadvantage of percutaneous management is that the integrity of the malignant urothelium is breached. Tumour seeding through the percutaneous tract has been reported and the potential for this complication must be borne in mind (Oefelein & MacLennan, 2003). For these reasons, retrograde endoscopic surgery should always be considered or attempted whenever possible.

Procedure

The aim of access is to provide a direct route to the lesion using a large working sheath (30F) and rigid endoscopic instrumentation. It is advantageous if this is done through a lower pole puncture as it avoids the greater morbidity associated with upper pole/intercostal punctures. Lesions in the upper ureter are best served with an upper pole puncture.

Resection requires biopsy of the tumour with cup forceps and coagulation of the tumour base. A 24F resectoscope may be employed for large tumours. Large vascular tumours can be coagulated with the Nd:YAG laser. The base of the tumour may be coagulated with either the Bugbee or rollerball electrode, or the Nd:YAG or holmium laser.

After resection, a nephrostomy tube should be left in place for 2 to 4 days. If the tumour is difficult to resect and doubt remains about completion, a nephrostomy tube should remain in place for a second-look procedure in a week's time. The threshold for a second-look procedure should be low. If adjuvant therapy is planned, the nephrostomy tube should remain

Table 10.5 Indications for percutaneous management of upper tract TCC	
Location	Tumour inaccessible by flexi URS due to anatomy, e.g. lower pole tumours or infundibular stenosis
Size	Large intrarenal tumours (>1.5 cm)
Access	Situations where retrograde access may be difficult, e.g. in patients with urinary diversion

until this is complete. The key steps for percutaneous surgery are listed in Box 10.7.

Box 10.7 Percutaneous treatment of upper tract TCC: operative steps

(1) Cystoscopy
(2) Insertion of ureteric catheter and retrograde ureteropyelography
(3) Patient positioning to prone oblique
(4) Percutaneous access
(5) Nephroscopy
(6) Tumour resection and ablation
(7) Insertion of nephrostomy tube
(8) +/− Second-look procedure
(9) +/− Retrograde adjuvant therapy

COMPLICATIONS OF PERCUTANEOUS MANAGEMENT

The major and minor complications of percutaneous resection of upper tract TCC are similar to those for PCNL, albeit the prevalence of sepsis is lower. Extraluminal seeding of tumour is a rare yet devastating complication (Box 10.8). It is usually a manifestation of the aggressive nature of the underlying pathology (high-grade/stage disease), although it has been reported after resection of a grade 2 tumour, presenting as an erythematous skin papule

---

Box 10.8 Reducing the risk of extraluminal seeding

(1) Avoid resection of high-grade tumours
(2) Perform percutaneous access and tumour resection as a single-stage procedure
(3) Avoid multiple tracts
(4) Keep low intrarenal pelvic pressures (<40 cm height irrigation and use Amplatz sheath)
(5) Avoid lengthy post-operative nephrostomy drainage
(6) Consider post-operative radiotherapy to the tract

---

over the scar (Oefelein & MacLennan, 2003). These concerns have led some to advocate using sterile water as the irrigant of choice because of its cytolytic effects. However, the potential for dilutional hyponatraemia has prevented this from becoming a popular choice. Some centres routinely give postoperative radiotherapy to the tract using iridium wire brachytherapy or external beam radiation (Mills et al., 2001). Failure of the tract to heal with a persisting urinary cutaneous fistula is a possible complication of this radiation therapy.

ADJUVANT TOPICAL IMMUNOTHERAPY / CHEMOTHERAPY

Topical immunological and chemotherapeutic agents may be used after retrograde or antegrade endoscopic resection (Table 10.6). The evidence of their value is not as robust compared to their role in the management of lower tract TCC. This is due to the limited number of patients with upper tract TCC treated endoscopically and discrepancies in patient selection between studies. Nevertheless, the number of studies indicating the efficacy and safety of topical adjuvant therapy, especially Bocillus Calnette-Guerin (BCG) therapy and mitomycin C, outnumbers studies that cast doubt on their role. With the propensity of TCC for polychronotropism and concern of extraluminal seeding after percutaneous treatment, the logical role of topical adjuvant therapy cannot be discounted. Although a clear survival advan-

Table 10.6 Adjuvant topical chemo/immunotherapy		
	Retrograde therapy	*Antegrade therapy*
Timing	Can be immediately after URS	1 to 2 weeks after percutaneous resection
Instillation method	Bladder instillation and Trendelenberg position with ureteral catheter/stent	Gravity drainage via nephrostomy tube (no more than 20–30 cm height)
	Period of exposure no more than 1 hour	
Complications	BCG: persistent pyrexia (5%), granulomatous change of kidney (25%), sepsis	
	Mitomycin C: toxic agranulocytosis	

tage of adjuvant therapy has not been proven, a reduction in the recurrence rate by at least a half is possible (Martinez-Pineiro et al., 1996).

BCG and mitomycin C are the most widely used agents (Box 10.9). They should not be used in the presence of ongoing haematuria or infection. They are well tolerated and safe with no detrimental effect on renal function. Mitomycin C has fewer side-effects compared to BCG (Table 10.6). Other agents such as interferon-α, 5-fluorouracil and thiotepa have been investigated, but with lower efficacy compared to either BCG or mitomycin C (Martinez-Pineiro et al., 1996).

> **DO!** Rule out obstruction and extravasation before adjuvant treatment. Maintain low urothelial pressures during instillation to reduce systemic absorption

BCG or mitomycin C may be given by retrograde administration through a bladder catheter whilst the patient is in Trendelenberg with an indwelling ureteral stent or catheter. This method is not as reliable as antegrade instillation through a nephrostomy tube. Patients with ileal conduits or known reflux can easily be treated via a bladder or conduit Foley catheter.

RECURRENCE AND SURVIVAL

Around 80% of patients who embark upon endoscopic surgery can expect to preserve their renal unit (Elliott et al., 2001). Recurrence may occur anywhere within the remaining ipsilateral and contralateral urothelium, including the bladder, prostatic urethra and penile urethra. The most important predictive factors for recurrence are tumour grade and stage (Box 10.10).

Box 10.9 Adjuvant therapy: indications

- Concomitant CIS
- High grade (2/3) tumours
- Large tumours
- Multiple tumours
- Residual tumours
- Post-percutaneous surgery

Box 10.10 Risk factors for recurrence

- CIS
- High grade
- High stage
- Tumour multiplicity
- Tumour size >1.5 cm

Overall, results from endoscopic resection of grade 1 and 2 tumours show comparable survival benefit when compared to radical surgery series (Lee et al., 1999). Patients who follow a strict surveillance protocol should find grade and disease progression is rare.

DO! Life-long endoscopic lower and upper tract surveillance is mandatory because of the high incidence of recurrence

---

Recurrence in the contralateral ureter is low (2–4%). The bladder is the most common site for recurrence and up to 40% of patients will develop bladder TCC (Tawfiek and Bagley, 1997). The impact of a previous history of bladder TCC on recurrence is debatable. Some studies have shown previous bladder TCC to be a risk factor (Keeley et al., 1997b; Martinez-Pineiro et al., 1996) whilst others have found neither superficial nor invasive bladder TCC to be a risk factor (Palou et al., 2004).

The overall recurrence rates in the upper tract from published series average around 30–40% for both ureteroscopy and percutaneous treatment. Grade 2 and 3 tumours have considerably higher recurrence rates (Table 10.7). Published mean time to recurrence after percutaneous treatment ranges from 11 to 48 months (Mills et al., 2001). Similar values have been obtained for ureteroscopic treatment; in a recent study of 21 patients with a 6-year mean follow-up, the mean time to recurrence was 7 months (Elliot et al., 2001).

The majority of upper tract recurrences occur in the proximity of the original tumour (Chen et al., 2000), which raises the question whether these tumours are small synchronous tumours missed the first time round. Factors that do not have any impact on the recurrence rate include the location of the primary lesion removed (intrarenal or ureteric) (Tawfiek & Bagley, 1997; Keeley et al., 1997b) and the method of resection (laser or electrosurgery) employed (Martinez-Pineiro et al., 1996).

Table 10.7 Recurrence and 5-year survival

	URS		Percutaneous	
	Recurrence rate[1] (%)	5 year survival[2] (%)	Recurrence rate[3] (%)	5-year survival[4] (%)
Grade 1	29	100	18	100
Grade 2	57	80	33	96
Grade 3	60	60	50	64

[1] Keeley et al., 1997: 38 pts, mean follow-up 35 mths.

[2] Elliott et al 1996: 37 pts, mean follow-up 60 mths.

[3] Jarrett et al., 1995: 30 pts, mean follow-up 55 mths.

[4] Liatsikos et al., 2001: 69 pts, mean follow-up 49 mths.

SURVEILLANCE

Surveillance must be life-long with patients willing to submit to a regular protocol before agreeing to endoscopic management. As there are no published guidelines on the optimal interval and choice of tests for surveillance of upper tract TCC, practices vary from centre to centre. A factor that is often forgotten when deciding a protocol is the patient's quality of life and the anxiety of having extra procedures. Therefore surveillance protocols must balance this aspect of the disease along with the potential morbidity and cost of further procedures with the desired aim of avoiding disease recurrence and progression. Table 10.8 outlines a protocol that is based on the work by Chen et al., 2000. Recurrent tumours should be regarded as new tumours and follow-up should start from the very beginning of the protocol.

Table 10.8 Suggested surveillance protocol

	Year 1	Year 2–3	Year 4 onwards
LA cystoscopy	3 monthly	3 monthly	6 monthly
Voided urine cytology	3 monthly	3 monthly	6 monthly
Cystoscopy, retrograde pyelography, selective cytology and ureteroscopy	3 monthly (until upper tract clear)	6 monthly	Annual
IVU	6 monthly	Annual	Annual

Of course, patients with severe medical problems cannot be expected to follow strict schedules.

Voided urine cytology should be combined with ureteroscopy and selective upper tract urine cytology/biopsy for surveillance in all patients. Chen et al. (2000) found ureteroscopy had a sensitivity of 93% and a specificity of 65%, and was much more accurate in detecting recurrence compared to retrograde pyelography (sensitivity 72%, specificity 85%) and bladder cytology (sensitivity 50%, specificity 100%). It is a point of debate whether ureteroscopic surveillance should be lifelong.

IVU and retrograde pyelography cannot be solely relied upon for detecting upper tract recurrence. During surveillance of 38 patients (mean follow-up 35 months), Keeley and colleagues found that retrograde pyelography failed to detect 75% of recurrent tumours which were subsequently diagnosed after ureteroscopy (Keeley et al., 1997b). The role of the IVU is to exclude cancer in the contralateral renal unit.

CONCLUSIONS/FUTURE TRENDS

The development of miniaturised endoscopes and ancillary equipment has made access to the upper tracts relatively straightforward with limited morbidity. This has allowed diagnostic ureterorenoscopy to be the investigation of choice for suspected upper tract TCC. The ability to perform intraluminal therapy has extended the endoscopic role into treatment of these conditions. Steadily the indication for treatment has evolved and extended such that low-grade tumours can be conservatively treated with good oncological control and renal preservation. However, poorly differentiated tumours and CIS remain a challenge that has not been overcome.

Certainly the endoscopic advances witnessed in the lower tract treatment of TCC over the past 30 years are being increasingly employed in the upper tract. It is more than likely that the endoscopic management of these tumours will develop further with a consequent reduction in the need for radical excision of the tumour being gained. The increase in the elderly population, many of whom have significant concomitant co-morbidities, will increase the role of endoscopic management in the future.

REFERENCES

Chen G, El-Gabry EA, Bagley DH. Surveillance of upper urinary tract transitional cell carcinoma: the role of ureteroscopy, retrograde pyelography, cytology and urinalysis. J Urol 2000; 164: 1901–4

Dodd LG, Johnston WW, Robertson CN, Layfield LJ. Endoscopic brush cytology of the upper urinary tract. Evaluation of its efficacy and potential limitations in diagnosis. Acta Cytol 1997; 41: 377–84

Elliott DS, Blute ML, Patterson DE, Bergstralh EJ, Segura JW. Long-term follow-up of endoscopically treated upper urinary tract transitional cell carcinoma. Urology 1996; 47: 819–25

Elliott DS, Segura JW, Lightner D, Patterson DE, Blute ML. Is nephroureterectomy necessary in all cases of upper tract transitional cell carcinoma? Long-term results of conservative endourologic management of upper tract transitional cell carcinoma in individuals with a normal contralateral kidney. Urology 2001; 58: 174–8

Hendin BN, Streem SB, Levin HS, Klein EA, Novick AC. Impact of diagnostic ureteroscopy on long-term survival in patients with upper tract transitional cell carcinoma. J Urol 1999; 161: 783–5

Jarrett TW, Sweetser PM, Weiss GH, Smith AD. Percutaneous management of transitional cell carcinoma of the renal collecting system: 9-year experience. J Urol. 1995; 154: 1629–35

Keeley FX, Kulp DA, Bibbo M, McCue PA, Bagley DH. Diagnostic accuracy of ureteroscopic biopsy in upper tract transitional cell carcinoma. J Urol 1997a; 157: 33–7

Keeley FX Jr, Bibbo M, Bagley DH. Ureteroscopic treatment and surveillance of upper urinary tract transitional cell carcinoma. J Urol 1997b; 157: 1560–5

Keeley FX Jr, Bibbo M, McCue PA, Bagley DH. Use of p53 in the diagnosis of upper-tract transitional cell carcinoma. Urology 1997; 49: 181–6

Lee BR, Jabbour ME, Marshall FF, Smith AD, Jarrett TW. 13-year survival comparison of percutaneous and open nephroureterectomy approaches for management of transitional cell carcinoma of renal collecting system: equivalent outcomes. J Endourol 1999; 13: 289–94

Liatsikos EN, Dinlenc CZ, Kapoor R, Smith AD. Transitional-cell carcinoma of the renal pelvis: ureteroscopic and percutaneous approach. J Endourol 2001; 15: 377–83

Martinez-Pineiro JA, Garcia Matres MJ, Martinez-Pineiro L. Endourological treatment of upper tract urothelial carcinomas: analysis of a series of 59 tumors. J Urol 1996; 156: 377–85

Mills IW, Laniado ME, Patel A. The role of endoscopy in the management of patients with upper urinary tract transitional cell carcinoma. BJU Int 2001; 87: 150–62

Oefelein MG, MacLennan G. Transitional cell carcinoma recurrence in the nephrostomy tract after percutaneous resection. J Urol 2003; 170: 521

Palou J, Piovesan LF, Huguet J, et al. Percutaneous nephroscopic management of upper urinary tract transitional cell carcinoma: recurrence and long-term followup. J Urol 2004; 172: 66–9

Rassweiler JJ, Schulze M, Marrero R, et al. Laparoscopic nephroureterectomy for upper urinary tract transitional cell carcinoma: is it better than open surgery? Eur Urol 2004; 46: 690–7

Tawfiek ER, Bagley DH. Upper-tract transitional cell carcinoma. Urology 1997; 50: 321–9

Zincke H, Aguilo JJ, Farrow GM, Utz DC, Khan AU. Significance of urinary cytology in the early detection of transitional cell cancer of the upper urinary tract. Urol 1976; 116: 781–3

SUGGESTED FURTHER READING

Chew BH, Pautler SE, Denstedt JD. Percutaneous management of upper-tract transitional cell carcinoma. J Endourol 2005; 19: 658–63

11. ENDOUROLOGICAL COMPLICATIONS AND THEIR MANAGEMENT

Complications following endoscopic or percutaneous renal surgery are classified as either major (life-threatening and requiring operative or radiological intervention) or minor (adequately managed with non-operative measures). They may occur during surgery, or in the early (1–7 days) or late (>7 days) post-operative period (see Table 11.1). For percutaneous renal stone surgery the major and minor complication rates are 2–4% and 10–25%, respectively (Lee et al., 1987). The overall complication rate after ureteroscopic stone surgery is 10–20%, with a major complication rate of 0–4% (Johnson & Pearle, 2004).

Table 11.1 Complications following percutaneous renal and ureteroscopic surgery

	Percutaneous renal surgery	Ureterorenoscopy
Intra-operative	Bleeding, loss of access, pelvic perforation, irrigation-related, abdominal organ injury, hydropneumothorax, equipment malfunction and instrument breakage	Avulsion, intussception, perforation, extravasation, submucosal tunnelling, mucosal abrasion and bleeding, thermal injury, equipment malfunction and instrument breakage, failure to progress
Early post-operative	Sepsis, pyrexia, bleeding, leaking misplaced nephrostomy tube, ureteric obstruction, retained stone, perinephric collection	Sepsis, infection, colic due to clot retention or oedema, retained fragment
Late post-operative	Infundibular stenosis, AV fistula, retained stone	Ureteric stricture, mucosal intraperitoneal fragments

SEPSIS

The incidence of sepsis (as defined in Box 11.1) after endoscopic stone manipulation in the upper urinary tract is 0.5–1.5% (Segura et al., 1985 O'Keefe et al., 1993). Out of 700 percutaneous or endoscopic stone procedures, O'Keefe et al. found that 1.3% of patients developed severe sepsis and 0.8% died. The severe sepsis rate after percutaneous nephrostomy insertion is 2%, although this is under 1% if daytime procedures are examined (Lewis & Patel, 2004). Additional clinical features of sepsis are listed in Box 11.2.

Box 11.1 Sepsis/severe sepsis/septic shock

Sepsis	Severe sepsis	Septic shock
A systemic inflammatory response to infection with evidence of two of the following four criteria:	Sepsis with dysfunction of one or more organs (or hypoperfusion or hypotension)	Severe sepsis that results in hypotension (systolic < 90 mmHg) unresponsive to fluid resuscitation
(1) Fever (>38°C) or hypothermia (<36°C)		
(2) Tachycardia (pulse rate > 90)		
(3) Tachypnoea (respiratory rate >20)		
(4) High (>12 000 mcl) or low (<4000 mcl) white cell count		

Box 11.2 More clinical features of sepsis

Temperature: sensation of cold (chills), shivering and rigors
Skin: may be warm and flushed, or pale and cool
Central nervous system: lethargy, disorientation, agitation, confusion
Serum analyses: coagulopathy, thrombocytopenia

Severe sepsis and septic shock

If unchecked, sepsis will proceed to severe sepsis and septic shock. Severe sepsis and septic shock can lead to multiple organ dysfunction syndrome (MODS), with a mortality approaching 70%.

Sepsis should be recognised early and resuscitation immediate. Bacteraemia or endotoxaemia stimulates cytokine release and initiates an inflammatory cascade that can result in coagulopathy, and disseminated intravascular coagulation (DIC) is almost universal in severe sepsis. Patients who develop sepsis should be jointly managed with the critical care team.

Sepsis and stone surgery

Stones, especially infection stones (struvite and calcium apatite) contain bacteria and endotoxins (cell wall protein of gram-negative bacteria). Endoscopic or percutaneous stone surgery may result in bacteraemia or endotoxaemia, or both.

TIP! Severe sepsis is likely to occur within the first 6 hours after a procedure

---

Pyrexia

Post-operative pyrexia occurs in 2 to 6% of patients after URS surgery (Johnson & Pearle, 2004). Mild pyrexia after PCNL is common, especially if the operation is on infection stones. The duration of surgery and amount of irrigation fluid are significant risk factors for post-operative pyrexia after PCNL (Troxel & Low, 2002). Box 11.3 lists causes of persistent pyrexia after PCNL. Post-operative antibiotics after non-complicated PCNL in the presence of sterile pre-operative mid-stream urine cultures are not warranted (Dogan et al., 2002).

Management of sepsis

The risk of sepsis depends upon the presence of various factors: type of stone (infection stone, impacted stone), complexity and length of operation, instrumentation used, irrigation pressure and patient factors (diabetes mellitus, poor renal function).

Management involves controlling the source of infection, instituting appropriate antibiotic therapy and immediate volume resuscitation with cardiopulmonary support.

Box 11.3 Causes of persistent pyrexia after PCNL

- Infection
- Ureteric obstruction
- Perinephric collection (urine/blood)
- Atelectasis/pneumonia – inadequate pain relief after supracostal puncture
- Pleural effusion – leaked irrigant after supracostal puncture

---

Controlling source of infection

During stone surgery, the best safeguard in controlling the source of infection is to adopt measures that limit the potential of bacteraemia and endotoxaemia. Antibiotic prophylaxis and surgical technique that avoids excessive stone manipulation reduces the risk of sepsis. Particular care must be taken with the staghorn calculus as it harbours many gram-negative bacteria (McAleer et al., 2002). Table 11.2 lists steps to take to minimise sepsis during percutaneous renal surgery.

Table 11.2 Methods to limit infection during antegrade and retrograde endoscopic surgery

Antibiotics
- Culture-specific antibiotic regime, 2-week pre-operative course, and continued until post-operative tubes/catheters are removed for:
  - (a) Infected calculi
  - (b) Pyrexia
  - (c) Symptoms of infection

Percutaneous access
- Obtain direct calyceal puncture
- Obtain clearance with minimum number of tracts

Instrumentation
- Larger endoscope for better visibility

Table 11.2 *continued*

- Clear stones as quickly as possible
- Keep amount of time spent on intracorporeal lithotripsy to minimum required

Irrigation

- Open low-pressure system (Amplatz sheath) to reduce extravasation of irrigant
- Avoid high-pressure irrigation and overdistension of collecting system (higher intrarenal pressures lead to bacteraemia)
- Abandon procedure early if poor views or perforation

Drainage

- Ensure adequate external or internal post-operative urinary drainage

Ureterorenoscopy (URS)

- Antibiotic prophylaxis should be given routinely for URS stone surgery
- Patients with positive urine cultures are at particular risk of sepsis, and require a post-operative course of culture specific antibiotics

DO! Maintain a low-pressure system by using a bladder catheter (Jacks) or use a ureteric catheter or ureteric access sheath to drain the collecting system for retrograde renal surgery

Instituting appropriate antibiotic therapy

Early administration of parenteral antibiotics can improve the likelihood of survival from septic shock. Antibiotics should cover gram-negative bacteria and mixed organisms. We use augmentin and gentamicin; a third- or fourth-generation cephalosporin is administered in the presence of poor renal function or penicillin allergy.

DO! Obtain blood for culture and sensitivity before administering antibiotics when sepsis is suspected

Volume resuscitation and cardiopulmonary support

Fluid resuscitation should be commenced at the earliest sign of sepsis. Prompt management can be the difference between life and death. Fever and chills are the earliest warning signs of sepsis. Rigors usually herald a more severe infectious process. Hypothermia is a worse prognostic sign than fever.

Initially a fluid challenge of 500–1000 ml crystalloid should be given (the rate should be adjusted for patients with congestive heart failure). Vigorous fluid resuscitation with 2–3 l of crystalloid (Hartmann's solution or 0.9% saline) over the first hour should be given if haemodynamic changes are present; colloid may also be added. If the patient is anaemic (<7.0 g/dl or <9.0 g/dl if ischaemic heart disease present) or coagulopathic then packed cells, fresh frozen plasma and platelets should be administered accordingly. Management should be in the critical care unit where invasive vascular monitoring should be instituted. If hypotension persists despite adequate volume resuscitation (septic shock), then ionotropic and vasoconstricting agents will be necessary.

IRRIGATION-RELATED COMPLICATIONS

Intravasation

Absorption of intra-operative irrigant fluid during percutaneous renal surgery may lead to sepsis, fluid/electrolyte overload and hypothermia. On average, patients can absorb 0.5–1 l of fluid during percutaneous renal surgery. In the majority, the fluid is absorbed with no ill effects. However, patients with compromised cardiorespiratory status may be at risk and will need careful monitoring.

Normal saline is the irrigant solution of choice for all endoscopic surgery unless diathermy is necessary, in which case a non-ionic solution will be necessary. Systemic fluid absorption can occur through pyelovenous lymphatic backflow, pyelotubular backflow and forniceal rupture or collecting system perforation, especially when intrarenal pressure is above 20–30 mmHg. Increased intrarenal pressure also occurs when irrigation outflow is restricted because of a narrow infundibulum or when the sheath is positioned incompletely within the collecting system (Troxel & Low, 2002). Table 11.3 lists the factors that can increase irrigation related complications.

Table 11.3 Factors increasing risk of irrigation related complications

Factor	Note
Operative time	Fluid absorption of greater than 1 l occurs when the irrigation fluid volume exceeds 10 l, and total irrigation time is greater than 30 minutes (Malhotra et al.)
Temperature of fluid	Warm fluids must always be used to avoid hypothermia
Bleeding or perforation of pelvicalyceal wall	Increases fluid absorption Operative time should be limited
Supracostal punctures	Risk of pleural fluid collection and effusion
Type of irrigating solution	Normal saline should always be used, however care must be taken when using glycine for electrosurgery. Excess amounts can lead to TUR syndrome (hyponatraemia, confusion, bradycardia, hypertension and vomiting)

Extravasation

Extravasation of irrigant fluid during PCNL may cause injury to surrounding retroperitoneal structures. Large intraperitoneal extravasation may cause ileus and rarely peritonitis. During ureteroscopy a large perforation may cause significant fluid absorption as the retroperitoneum absorbs fluid well. Rarely, periureteral and perirenal fibrosis can follow large volume fluid extravasation.

INJURIES TO COLLECTING SYSTEM

PCNL

Minor injury to the collecting system is not uncommon, and extravasation occurs in up to 10% of cases. Most resolve on nephrostomy or ureteric drainage, although large volume extravasation will result in urinoma. More worrisome is pelvic perforation due to medial extension of the tract or trauma from instrumentation (Figure 11.1). The operation should be terminated if perirenal structures are visualised through the nephroscope. A ureteric stent and nephrostomy tube should be left in place until watertight healing is confirmed. Undiagnosed perforation can lead to abdominal

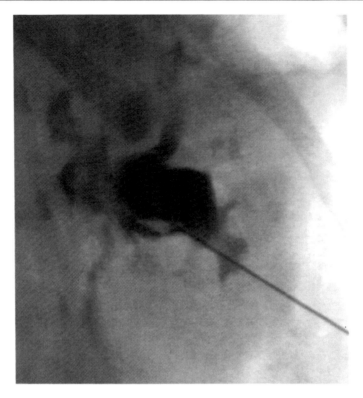

Figure 11.1 Image taken during nephrostomy insertion showing extravasation of contrast from a pelvic perforation.

distension, deteriorating fluid balance and sepsis. Significant pelvic perforations may rarely require delayed open or laparoscopic repair. Injury to renal lymphatics can lead to chyluria.

URS

Persistent pyrexia, abdominal distension and ileus after ureteroscopy suggest a retroperitoneal urinoma (incidence 0.5 to 1%). Management is percutaneous drainage and ensuring urinary diversion, either via a stent or nephrostomy. A swinging pyrexia may indicate abscess formation.

URETERIC INJURIES

The type of ureteric injury encountered during ureteroscopy is specific to the pathology being treated (stone, TCC), the ureteric location (distal vs proximal

ureter) and the instrumentation used (flexible vs rigid endoscopy, Lithoclast®
vs laser lithotripsy, basket vs forcep retrieval). Perforation and avulsion are
more likely to occur in the thin-walled proximal ureter. The distal ureter has
a thick wall, and therefore submucosal tunnelling is more likely in this location. Complications of ureteroscopy are associated with increased operative
time, treating stones in the kidney, decreased surgeon experience and use of
semirigid endoscopy over flexible endoscopy (Schuster et al., 2001).

Major complications

Avulsion

This is a nightmare scenario. Fortunately, its incidence in current practice is
extremely rare (<0.1%). It is usually a result of aggressive basket removal
of an impacted stone in the mid or proximal ureter, where the ureteral wall
is much thinner, or by ignoring the age old adage 'don't push'. Ignoring the
strong resistance encountered when withdrawing the basket will result in a
catastrophe that can be avoided (see Box 11.4).

Box 11.4. How to avoid avulsion

- When navigating the ureter, make sure the whole lumen is visualised
  at all times
- Ensure walls of ureter move in relation to the endoscope during
  manipulations
- If resistance is met, do not force through – dilate or come back
- Always fragment stones to size of the narrowest point of the ureter
- If you anticipate trouble, use a pronged grasper instead of a basket to
  remove stone
- Do not basket proximal ureteral stones
- Never force a basket down
- If stone and basket are stuck, take basket apart and perform
  lithotripsy to fragment the stone in the basket

If avulsion is recognised at the time of surgery, immediate open or laparoscopic surgical repair can be offered if the surgeon is confident in reconstruc-
tive surgery and not too shaken up by the traumatic experience! If this is not
possible, insertion of a nephrostomy tube will avoid significant extravasation

and bide time for a delayed repair. Ureteroneocystostomy, Boari flap, end-to-end anastomosis, ileal interposition and nephrectomy are the options available depending on the location and severity of the injury. A partial avulsion may be treated by either retrograde or antegrade ureteric stenting for 4 to 6 weeks, but the incidence of subsequent stricture is significant.

Intussusception

This is a partial thickness circumferential injury of the ureteral lumen which usually occurs due to aggressive basket retrieval of stone. The ureteral lumen develops an invagination of mucosa, and the ureter distal to the injury is devitalised. Late complication is ureteral stricture or necrosis and open or laparoscopic repair may be necessary.

Stricture

The incidence of ureteric stricture after URS is 0.5%. Stricture is associated with ureteral perforation, prolonged impacted calculi (ischaemic ureter), excessive instrumentation leading to ureteral trauma and large calibre instruments. Patients at risk of developing stricture will require follow-up imaging to document drainage and exclude silent obstruction. Stricture of the PUJ or upper ureter may also occur after PCNL (Figure 11.2) from impacted calculi or from traumatic access, dilation or endoscopy. In addition, previous radiotherapy or surgery or prolonged periods of calculus obstruction can lead to stricture formation.

Minor complications

Perforation

This is an uncommon complication of ureteroscopy. The perforation may be recognised during surgery or diagnosed after a retrograde ureterogram. It may be a result of guidewire passage, intracorporeal lithotripsy or endoscopic trauma. Modern series show an incidence of <2%.

If recognised early, irrigation must be reduced to avoid massive extravasation into the retroperitoneum and the operation terminated as soon as possible. Conservative treatment with a short course of antibiotics and ureteric stenting for 3 to 6 weeks is all that is required in the majority. A perforation in the upper ureter may also occur during PCNL when removing stones, attempting antegrade stenting or inserting a drainage catheter. Treatment is as above with or without covering nephrostomy drainage.

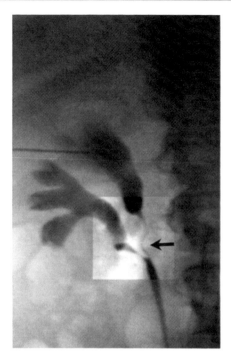

Figure 11.2 Ureteric stricture that occurred after PCNL. The arrow points to the narrowed area that extends into the upper and lower pole infundibula. This responded well to percutaneous balloon dilatation.

Mucosal abrasion and bleeding

This is less of a problem with the introduction of smaller calibre endoscopes. However, repeated contact between the scope and the ureteral walls can result in mucosal abrasion and oedema. Bleeding may ensue that reduces visibility. Most bleeding is minor and self-limiting. A ureteric stent should be inserted if there is any concern of clot retention. A ureteral access sheath can be useful if repeated insertions of the scope are envisaged.

Submucosal tunnelling

Ancillary instrumentation and even the endoscope can perforate and travel through the submucosal layer, especially in the distal ureter. Most false passages are minor and may be left alone, but larger ones will warrant stenting for a few weeks to reduce stricture formation.

> **DON'T!** If you feel any resistance whilst passing the guidewire then stop. It may have gone up the submucosal space

Thermal injury

Injury to the ureter from the heat generated by intracorporal lithotriptors (laser, USL, EHL) can cause fibrosis and stricture formation.

> **DO!** Keep the laser fibre parallel with the ureteral wall to minimise mucosal contact

Colic

Post-operative pain is not uncommon. Persistent pain and pyrexia in the absence of a ureteric stent should alert the clinician to the possibility of ureteral obstruction from either oedema, blood clot or retained stone fragment. Imaging should diagnose the level and degree of obstruction, which can be managed by ureteric stenting or nephrostomy drainage.

CALCULI EXTRUSION

Stone fragments expelled into the retroperitoneal or perinephric space should not be retrieved. The fragment position should be identified on radiography and patient education and documentation in the notes are essential to avoid future confusion and unnecessary intervention. Stone granuloma due to fragments propulsed into the submucosa appear as a bulge in the ureteral wall. These can lead to stricture and can be safely deroofed with the holmium laser.

EQUIPMENT MALFUNCTION AND INSTRUMENT BREAKAGE

Equipment failure during a procedure is all too common and invariably unexpected. The immediate availability of a second sterilised set of endoscopic equipment is vital for patient safety. Faulty kit should not be used and if an alternative kit is not available in a reasonable period of time the procedure should be abandoned at that stage.

> **DON'T!** If faulty equipment cannot be exchanged the operation should not proceed

COMPLICATIONS SPECIFIC TO PCNL

Bleeding after PCNL

Blood loss after PCNL is common. Transfusion is required in <5–15% of cases (Lee et al., 1987) and is more common with prolonged operating times, multiple punctures and larger stone volumes (especially staghorn calculi). Bleeding may be intra-operative, early (2–7 days) or late (>7 days) (Table 11.4). Most intra-operative bleeding is tract-related (Figure 11.3) and can be minimised by following anatomical principles of access.

While the sheath is being placed, care must be taken to avoid puncturing the renal pelvis which is rich in blood vessels. Rough instrumentation can cause damage to blood vessels within the pelvicalyceal wall. Severe haemorrhage necessitating angiographic intervention is rare (0.8%) (Kessaris et al., 1995). Initial measures include nephrostomy tube clamping and tract balloon inflation and, if they are not successful, proceed to angiography and embolisation (Figure 11.4). Very rarely open exploration may be necessary.

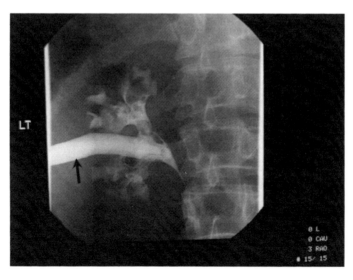

Figure 11.3 *This image shows clot in the collecting system from track bleeding. A tamponade balloon catheter has been inserted (arrow).*

(a)

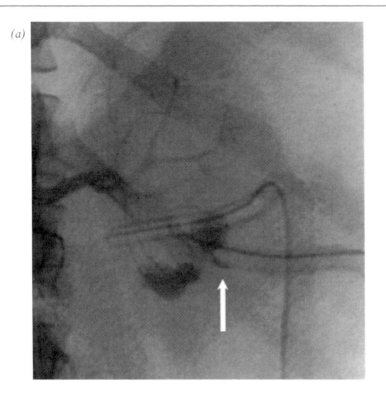

(b)

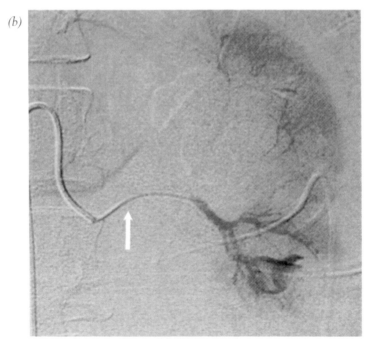

(c)

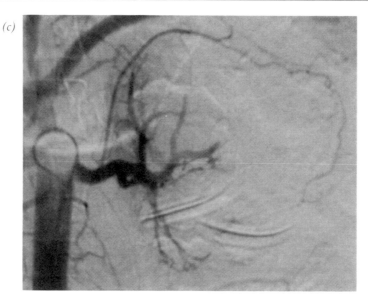

Figure 11.4 Three images showing a major post-PCNL haemorrhage that required urgent angiograhy (6 hours post-PCNL). (a) Shows an actively bleeding lobar branch (arrow); (b) shows superselective catherisation (arrow) of this branch and (c) is the post-embolisation image.

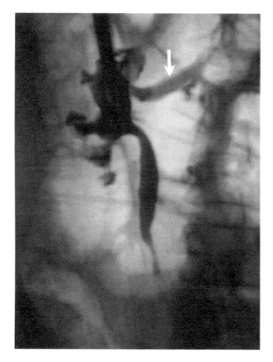

Figure 11.5 Post-PCNL nephrostogram shows venous tear (arrow) as the source of the continued post-PCNL bleed; this closed spontaneously.

Table 11.4 Bleeding after PCNL

Timing	Cause	Management
Intra-operative	Tract-related	Most bleeding is short-lived and is tamponaded by the sheath when its tip is in the collecting system
		Persistent bleeding can be controlled by clamping a large bore nephrostomy tube (tamponade) or inserting a Kaye nephrostomy tamponade balloon (Cook Urological)
Early post-operative	Venous (dark) from the track	Usually the nephrostomy tube has retreated into the track and repositioning it into the renal pelvis stops the bleeding.
		A nephrostogram may show a venous tear (Figure 11.5), which if large enough is treated by prolonged tamponade with the nephrostomy catheter (10–14 days)
Immediate or early post-operative bleeding	Arterial bleeding. May occur later on due to bleeding from an arteriovenous fistula or pseudoaneurysm	Arterial bleeding can cause immediate and dramatic haemorrhage.

Early or late bleeding leading to haemodynamic instability necessitates resuscitation and urgent angiography with a view to selective embolisation |

Injury to adjacent organs

Lung and pleura

Pneumothorax, hydrothorax and haemothorax can occur at varying rates depending upon the percutaneous approach and the operative side. The right chest wall has a greater risk of injury than the left side. Intrathoracic complications are greater with supracostal access compared to subcostal punctures (Figure 11.6).

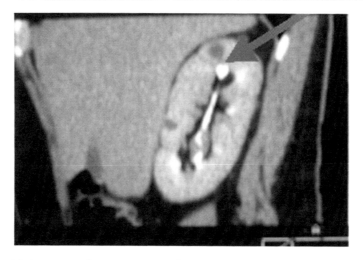

Figure 11.6 A sagittal reconstruction of a CT scan showing how upper pole access can breach the pleura and lung.

A prospective analysis of supra-12th rib access showed the overall chest complication rate to be 11% (Gupta et al., 2002). Intrathoracic complications from a supra-11th rib access are considerably higher. A retrospective analysis of 300 percutaneous procedures showed the chest complication rate from a supra-11th rib access to be 23.1% compared to 1.4% for supra-12th and 0.5% for infra-12th rib access (Munver et al., 2001).

DO! Get a post-operative CXR in recovery after a supracostal access

---

TIP! Watch out for patients with low O_2 saturation, tachypnoea or dyspnoea after a PCNL

Hydropneumothorax

Hydro/pneumothorax is the most common chest complication. Haemothorax is usually a result of intercostal artery injury. In one study, 38% of patients after PCNL had hydropneumothorax diagnosed on CT compared to only 8% diagnosed after postoperative CXR (Ogan et al., 2003). The majority are clinically insignificant, and intervention will only be required in those with symptoms (Figure 11.7). Chest fluoroscopy after

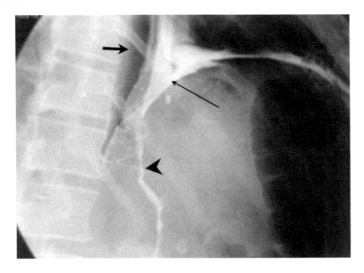

Figure 11.7 This nephrostogram shows a hydropneumothorax as a complication of intercostal PCNL (above the 12th rib). The arrowhead shows the fistulous track between the retroperitoneum and the pleura outlined by contrast, the short arrow points to the pneumothorax and the long arrow points to the hydrothorax.

PCNL may detect large effusions or pneumothoraces, allowing tube thoracostomy drainage in theatre whilst the patient is under anaesthesia.

Supracostal punctures

DO! When making a puncture stay above the upper border of the lower rib to avoid injury to the neurovascular bundle directly below the ribs
DO! Use a working sheath that is well fitted to the tract during surgery to minimise the size of a hydrothorax

---

Nephropleural fistulae

There should be a high index of suspicion for this complication after supra-costal punctures. Prolonged nephrostomy tube drainage (at least a week) should allow the fistula to close. Delayed nephropleural fistula may present 1 to 2 weeks after the nephrostomy tube has been removed with sudden onset tachypnoea. A nephrostogram will show communication between the collecting system and intrathoracic cavity. Treatment is drainage of the pleural effusion and ureteric stenting to divert urinary drainage until the pleural drainage has subsided.

Colon

Colonic injury is rare (reported rate 0.5%). At risk of injury are young thin adults and those with retrorenal or posteriorly displaced colon which are more common on the left side and in women. Intraperitoneal injuries may lead to peritonitis and require urgent open surgery. Fortunately the majority of injuries are extraperitoneal and can be managed conservatively (Box 11.5). During surgery if the sheath slips out of the kidney into the colon, gas or faeces may be seen coming out of the sheath, or diarrhoea may be noticed on table. Post-operative fever, pneumaturia or faecaluria should alert the clinician to this complication. Most injuries, however, are silent and presentation is delayed until faeces is noted coming out of the nephrostomy tube or contrast is seen draining into the colon on nephrostogram.

Box 11.5 Management of extraperitoneal colonic injury

- Remove nephrostomy tube
- Insert ureteric stent and urethral catheter
- Percutaneous drainage of pericolonic space
- Bowel rest: nil by mouth, antibiotics, nutrition

If extraperitoneal injury is recognised at the time of surgery, the nephrostomy tube may be exchanged for a catheter which is secured in the colon (colostomy tube). If the patient is stable, a second percutaneous access tract can be placed more medially and superior to the original site, through which nephrolithotomy can be performed.

Duodenum

Compared to colonic perforation, duodenal injury is less common. A large perforation of the pelvis or lower pole collecting system of the right kidney may extend into the second or third part of the duodenum. Management is conservative, similar to colonic injury, however nephroduodenal fistulae take longer to resolve.

Other organs

Splenic and liver injuries are extremely rare. The liver is more forgiving to injury, however splenic injuries are more likely to bleed and require operative intervention.

Infundibular stenosis after PCNL

The reported incidence of this late complication is 2%, with most occurring within the year of PCNL (Parsons et al., 2002). Risk factors are listed in Box 11.6. Significant stenosis may be associated with impaired renal function, and patients at risk will require careful radiographic follow-up.

Box 11.6 Risk factors for developing infundibular stenosis after PCNL

---

(1) Large stone burden
(2) Long operative time
(3) Multiple subsequent procedures (ESWL or PCNL)
(4) Prolonged nephrostomy tube drainage
(5) Upper pole punctures (Figure 11.2)

Kidney function post-PCNL

Although there may be some local scarring after PCNL, nuclear medicine studies have found no significant short- or long-term deterioration in renal function, even after PCNL in solitary kidneys.

REFERENCES

Dogan HS, Sahin A, Cetinkaya Y, et al. Antibiotic prophylaxis in percutaneous nephrolithotomy: prospective study in 81 patients. J Endourol 2002; 16: 649–53

Gupta R, Kumar A, Kapoor R, Srivastava A, Mandhani A. Prospective evaluation of safety and efficacy of the supracostal approach for percutaneous nephrolithotomy. BJU Int 2002; 90: 809–13

Johnson DB, Pearle MS. Complications of ureteroscopy. Urol Clin North Am 2004; 31: 157–71

Kessaris DN, Bellman GC, Pardalidis NP, Smith AG. Management of hemorrhage after percutaneous renal surgery. J Urol 1995; 153: 604–8

Lee WJ, Smith AD, Cubelli V, et al. Complications of percutaneous nephrolithotomy. Am J Roentgenol 1987; 148: 177–80

Lewis S, Patel U. Major complications after percutaneous nephrostomy – lessons from a department audit. Clin Radiol 2004; 59: 171–9

McAleer IM, Kaplan GW, Bradley JS, Carroll SF. Staghorn calculus endotoxin expression in sepsis. Urology 2002; 59: 601

Malhotra SK, Khaitan A, Goswami AK, et al. Monitoring of irrigation fluid absorption during percutaneous nephrolithotripsy: the issue of 1% ethanol as a marker. Anaesthesia 2001; 56: 1103–6

Munver R, Delvecchio FC, Newman GE, Preminger GM. Critical analysis of supracostal access for percutaneous renal surgery. J Urol 2001; 166: 1242–6

Ogan K, Corwin TS, Smith T, et al. Sensitivity of chest fluoroscopy compared with chest CT and chest radiography for diagnosing hydropneumothorax in association with percutaneous nephrostolithotomy. Urology 2003; 62: 988–92

O'Keefe NK, Mortimer AJ, Sambrook PA, Rao PN. Severe sepsis following percutaneous or endoscopic procedures for urinary tract stones. Br J Urol 1993; 72: 277–83

Parsons JK, Jarrett TW, Lancini V, Kavoussi LR. Infundibular stenosis after percutaneous nephrolithotomy. J Urol 2002; 167: 35–8

Schuster TG, Hollenbeck BK, Faerber GJ, Wolf JS Jr. Complications of ureteroscopy: analysis of predictive factors. J Urol 2001; 166: 538–40

Segura JW, Patterson DE, LeRoy AJ, et al. Percutaneous removal of kidney stones: review of 1,000 cases. J Urol 1985; 134: 1077–81

Troxel SA, Low RK. Renal intrapelvic pressure during percutaneous nephrolithotomy and its correlation with the development of postoperative fever. J Urol 2002; 168: 1348–51

SUGGESTED FURTHER READING

Gerspach JM, Bellman GC, Stoller ML, Fugelso P. Conservative management of colon injury following percutaneous renal surgery. Urology 1997; 49: 831–6

INDEX

Printed and bound by CPI Group (UK) Ltd, Croydon, CR0 4YY

23/10/2024

01777708-0002